QUESTIONS AND ANSWERS ABOUT

Callanetics

Is this book easy to follow?
Yes. The instructions for the exercises are simple and clear and accompanied with photographs to show how it's done.

Will I have to work hard at these exercises?
Yes, they are not easy—at first. But 1 hour of Callanetics is equal to 7 hours of more conventional exercise as far as muscle tone, stamina, and visible results are concerned.

How often do I have to do Callanetics?
One hour twice a week will get spectacular results. Once you have reached your perfect figure, maintenance can be reduced to 1 hour a week.

Do I have to start with a whole hour of exercise right at the beginning?
No. It is preferable to spread out the first hour over 4 days in 15-minute segments, until the exercises become easy enough for you to continue them for a full hour at a stretch.

Will I still see results if I exercise only 15 minutes a day?
Absolutely. The results are as visible as if you did them all at once. It just takes a little longer that way.

How did Callan Pinckney develop Callanetics?
The author is an ex-ballet dancer (classical) who spent years backpacking around the world. This kind of travel, plus the problem of a congenital back defect, caused a physical breakdown. To get her body back into shape she combined exercises that she learned in Europe with her own experimental innovations. She resculpted her figure while curing her problems and eventually opened a studio where she teaches these exercises. She has been featured in *Working Womar* and *Vogue* magazines.

Callanetics:
10 Years Younger
in 10 Hours

Callanetics: 10 Years Younger in 10 Hours

BY CALLAN PINCKNEY

with Sallie Batson

Photographs by Gary Moody

William Morrow and Company, Inc./New York

Library of Congress Cataloging in Publication Data

Pinckney, Callan.
   Callanetics: 10 years younger in 10 hours.

   1. Exercise. 2. Reducing exercises. 3. Physical
fitness. 4. Rejuvenation. 5. Youthfulness. 6. Pinckney,
Callan. I. Batson, Sallie. II. Moody, Gary. III. Title.
IV. Title: Ten years younger in ten hours with callan-
etics. V. Title: Callanetics.
RA781.P575 1984   646.7'5   84-6565
ISBN 0-688-03787-9

Printed in the United States of America

       24 25 26 27 28 29 30

BOOK DESIGN BY ABBY KAGAN

THIS BOOK IS DEDICATED:

—to my precious, darling mother, who faithfully massaged
my legs three hours a day for five years;
—to all the people around the world who were so
concerned for my safety, for without their kindnesses I
probably would have never made it home;
—and to my students who have taught me so much and
eased my readjustment into the American way of life.

SPECIAL CREDITS

Travel photos by whoever could aim the camera and push the button.

Medical Researcher: Michelle Dellapenta, R.N., C.N. II
Special Researcher: Valerie S. Brown

Sculptures by Edwina Sandys
Hair and Makeup by Lillian Cortez

Consultants: Mary Ann Castro, R.N.; New York City Police Sgt. John P. Codiglia, Mr. New York's Finest, State Body Building Champion in 1982 and 1983; Ellen M. Godowitz, M.Th.; Hiromichi Hayashi, M.C., P.C.; Kim Johnson; Dr. Laurie Langer; Dr. Pasquale A. Luongo; Dr. Patrick M. Luongo; Charles McCarroll; M.S.C., C.S.W.; Carl Bruno Menkel; Norman Miller Associates; Jacqueline I. Ross, R.P.T.; and Leonard Russell of the Sheridan Square Health Club.

Special Thanks to: Peggy Batson, Helen Mary Breen, Dianne Brooks, Lulu Buras, Irene Cara, Robert M. Cavallo, Dara Cohen, Susan Croft, Mark Dixon, Valdev Duggal, Mitch Douglas, Louise Duncan, Paula Fierman, Larry Finley, Barbara Friedlander, Pat Golbitz, Tina Jorgenson-Rubbo, Charles and Suzanne Lecht, Marie McGrath, Lynne Meena, Tanya Mendoza, Jane Pinckney Middleton, Lane Middleton, Page Middleton, Janet Milazzo, Alan Peseri, Joan Poole, Karl S. Sabo, Ray Steinberg, Elba Tanburino, Arlene Tarte, Tara Terrell, Neal Thompson, Anna Tipton, Lynn Tuttle, Jennifer Williams, to Jane Angus, who wrote the initial proposal, and, especially, to Ebba Olsen Thomson, my ballet teacher.

A NOTE OF CAUTION

Before beginning this, or any other, exercise program, it is advisable to obtain the approval and recommendations of your physican. While you're on this, or any, exercise program, it is advisable to visit your physician for periodic monitoring. This program is intended for adults in good health.

Contents

CHAPTER ONE

Who Is Callan Pinckney and Why Is She Writing This Book?

Callan Pinckney is not a celebrity, model, or movie star, nor is she a medical doctor with a string of degrees. She is a teacher, albeit unorthodox, of one of the most innovative exercise programs today. How she became a teacher is not so simple to explain. How she devised the program began somewhere between Savannah, Georgia, and Southeast Asia, sometime in the 1960s.

On paper, Callan's life looks like the figment of a fertile imagination, a scenario for a movie script:

A ninth-generation American Southern debutante, Callan hopped a freighter bound for Germany in 1961 and hitch-hiked around the world for the better part of ten years, completely missing the turbulent sixties in this country.

She shoveled snow in London, tracked migrating herds in Central Africa, painted the decks of a freighter as a member of its crew, sold peanuts table to table in a fashionable Tokyo rooftop restaurant, and taught British pronunciation to four hundred Chinese children in Hong Kong. These are but a few of her survival jobs.

Born with spinal curvatures (scoliosis and swayback), one hip higher than the other, and feet turned inward so severely that she wore leg braces to her waist for seven years of her childhood, Callan went on to study classical ballet for twelve years with a protégé of the legendary Michel Fokine.

Today she teaches exercise to diplomats and ambassadors, recording stars, actors and actresses, housewives, doctors, as well as to business and professional people of all sizes, shapes, and ages.

Callan was presented to Savannah society at the 1959 Debutante Cotillion. Her formal portrait shows her in an intricately beaded gown before a massive antique mirror. Within two years, she stepped through a looking glass of another sort and this traditional southern lifestyle was, for her, gone forever. ▲

Descended from the same Pinckney family that was instrumental in the founding of this country, especially South Carolina, even helping to draft the Constitution of the United States, Callan comes from a long line of special achievers. At the age of seventeen, Eliza Lucas Pinckney was single-handedly responsible for finding the process that made indigo the most profitable export crop of the colonies for more than thirty years until the American Revolution severed our relationship with the primary consumer, Great Britain. George Washington was a pallbearer at her funeral. Charles Cotesworth Pinckney, her son, negotiated the Pinckney Treaty of 1795 with France, laying the groundwork for the purchase, less than a decade later, of the entire Louisiana Territory.

The United States of America was not the first country that the Pinckneys helped to settle. They were with William the Conqueror at the Norman Invasion in 1066. A British noblewoman quipped to a contemporary Pinckney family historian: "My God, you Pinckneys cover the world!"

Callan's maternal ancestry contributes further to this colorful woman's spirit of adventure. These hearty souls—the Pfeiffers—trekked from the heart of the Pennsylvania Dutch territory, across the Oregon Trail, to settle in the Pacific Northwest.

Growing up in and around Savannah, Georgia, Callan was taught to be a proper Southern Lady, with all the trimmings, rebelling all the way. "I was suspended by almost every school I attended," she confesses. "I didn't want to be there. I was busy dreaming of being in foreign lands. I wanted to experience life and people, not read about them in books."

Despite her aversion to academic ventures, Callan completed two years of college. The final straw was when she spotted her hosts at a fraternity party spying through a peephole into the ladies' room. "If those boys were to be the future of our country, I didn't want any part of them," she recounts. "I sold my books and went back to Savannah."

Callan worked as a clerk in a department store, saving every penny and plotting her "getaway." This was a bit scandalous, considering her family's background, but she was not thinking of appearances: The sales job paid more than anything else she could find, and money was what she was after, keeping expenses to a minimum, saving the balance for her travels.

Her father had adamantly prohibited her going abroad until she completed her college education. Callan was equally adamant about going. "My father's telling me I couldn't live three months without his support was the first major challenge in my life."

Her Great Escape came when she threw her suitcase from a second-story window and climbed out after it, leaving her parents' home behind. Friends drove her to the depot where she caught a bus for Wilmington, North Carolina. There she boarded a freighter bound for Germany.

The year was 1961. There was little indication of what lay ahead for this country during the decade to follow. Kennedy was President. Everyone was singing about Camelot. Women wore skirts to go shopping and dressed up when they traveled by plane. Men had weekly haircuts, wore socks that matched their Madras sportscoats and oxford-cloth shirts, and opened doors and tipped their hats for ladies. The Love Generation and the antiwar movement were yet go to public.

Armed with little more than her passport, Callan Pinckney was off to see the world.

Arriving in Bremerhaven, West Germany, the petite brunette had no particular itinerary, just an insatiable curiosity that led her through Europe for almost a year. In Germany, she acquired a Volkswagen for a friend. This was to become her home to cut expenses.

Without work permits, Callan took odd jobs to supplement her savings. Her first winter in London, she shoveled snow and coal for what amounted to $3.36 for an eight-hour day. There was no central heating and Callan was not accustomed to the frigid temperatures. She lived on biscuits and jam, cookies, and quantities of starchy foods to insulate her body in fat. Before long, she weighed 129 pounds—quite a jump for someone who is only an inch over five-feet tall and whose previous top weight had been 105.

Hearing about Africa from people she met in London, Callan explored the possibilities of going there. She was unable to get the necessary travel permits in England, so she hitchhiked to Hamburg and secured papers there, returning briefly to London to tie up loose ends and to purchase the rucksack that was to be her "mobile home" for the next eight or nine years.

For a while Callan worked in Capetown for an advertising agency by day and as a waitress by night. She talked her way into most of the jobs she held during her travels, determined to learn whatever skills were necessary once she secured the position.

Her soft, cultured Southern accent was foreign to Callan's British and Afrikaans employers and co-workers. Consequently, she was asked to come to the office a half hour early every morning to be tutored in "proper English pronunciation." "I was quite insulted. I told them I spoke *modern* English, not Elizabethan," she laughs. Today, her accent is part American, part British, and all Callan. She is a verbal chameleon, reflecting the accents of those around her.

She spent almost a year in the bush of Central Africa. Part of this time she helped track animal migrations from place to place, leaving Zimbabwe, then Rhodesia, Zaire, then the Congo, and Kenya, when trouble began to brew.

Her survival instincts kept her body alive, but did not keep her fit and healthy. Her rapid weight gain in England had caused stretch marks on her hips. Her erratic, often inadequate, diet lead to malnutrition and three debilitating bouts of amoebic dysentery. ("I had diarrhea for eight years.") She dropped from a pudgy 129 to 78 pounds during the worst of these attacks. She was on Cyprus and had to be evacuated from the RAF Hospital there to make room for the wounded soldiers brought in from battle daily.

Callan further abused her body by doing menial labor to earn money and by carrying her backpack. Weighing almost as much as she did, it pulled her collar bones and strained her back and knees mercilessly.

For most of her odyssey, Callan lived among peasants, without any of the conveniences she had taken for granted all of her life. To this day she brushes her teeth without water. She usually wears a sweater or has one handy even in summer, remembering her fear of freezing for lack of clothing. "When I first returned to the States, I identified with the street people, the shopping bag ladies," she confides. "I wanted to know what they carried in their bags, if the contents resembled what I had carried."

In most of the countries where she lived or traveled, there was nothing written in English, not even signs on buildings. Callan tells that she had been living in New York for several years, following her travels abroad, wondering how people always knew the names of stores and streets. She had spent so much time in places where signs were unreadable that she had forgotten to look at them.

Callan maintained a detailed diary throughout her travels. As she left a country, she mailed a diary to her parents, making sure she could not be traced. "I never knew where I would be going next," she explains. "I went where the roads and rides took me. I didn't care where they went." As for her diaries: "To this day I haven't read them. I don't think I ever shall."

Much of this time she was alone, although sometimes she traveled with a Canadian girl whom she met early in her trip.

Callan planned to hitchhike from Johannesburg to Japan. She expected the trip to take about six months. It took seven years.

In Bombay, India, she was in an air raid. "I was walking down a street when a plane flew over and began shooting. I froze. Two men grabbed me and threw me into a doorway for cover. I hid my face in my arms and waited for the shooting to stop. When I looked up, I saw a hand with only three fingers next to me. I was lying next to a leper. One of my greatest fears while traveling the world was contracting that disease."

This prompted Callan to travel south to Ceylon. She and her Canadian companion, joined by an American girl who had been staying in the same place in Bombay, rode third class on the train to the border. Callan slept on luggage racks because the compartments, which had comfortable space for fifteen people, contained as many as sixty.

The trio missed the boat from India to Ceylon (now Sri Lanka) and had to wait a week for passage. To occupy their time, Callan introduced her American cohort to basic ballet. "That was the first time I noticed I could not do movements I had once been able to do so beautifully. I had no flexibility or extension. My muscles had no tone."

She did not understand why it hurt whenever she sat. Her behind had fallen so much that it was now on her hips. Sitting on her sweater to cushion her tailbone had become second nature. Sleeping with a rag between her knees to keep them from rubbing together was a necessity.

Newspapers and current events were no longer a part of Callan's life. Her day-to-day considerations were personal safety, drinkable water, clean food for survival, and finding a safe place to sleep.

Once Callan reached Japan, she recorded British voice-over tapes for advertising, wrote about her travels for a Japanese magazine, and modeled miniskirts. She also managed a bar and was responsible for hiring Western waitresses.

At that time, Callan was becoming increasingly aware of her body's need for care. Back in London, she began to work seriously on her body. This was a slow, painful process for someone who had become so run-down. Doctors advised her to have surgery on her travel-damaged knees and cautioned that her back would never recover. "I looked terrible and was in constant pain. I thought that if I had to hurt all the time, I might as well look good. I had no other choice."

When Callan returned to the United States, she appeared so emaciated and old that her mother fainted upon seeing her emerge from the plane.

Callan's first job upon returning to the United States in 1972 was at a New York City exercise salon. "I left there because I didn't approve of the way clients' bodies were being treated. I was told to change the way I had been instructed to teach the exercises, supposedly so we could handle more clients in the salon. The owner of the franchise prohibited my asking the women I worked with if they had back problems, yet my back hurt when I did some of the exercises. Other people might have been hurting as well. This was extremely upsetting for me. The salon's owner and I had studied this program from a woman who is a master in this field. I believed in my teacher's program, and, in all fairness to her and to myself, I could not continue the way things were going."

After leaving the salon, Callan experimented with other techniques, and the movements learned while studying ballet. "I found that if I felt back pain, I could simply shift my position as little as a fraction of an inch until my back no longer hurt. I got incredible results. I was determined not to do anything to start the back spasms again. I was amazed to see how strong and tight my body had become. My back had stopped hurting. I felt and looked as though I had been exercising for three hours a day for five years after only a few hours of these movements. I concluded that these delicate, precise movements are the key to successful exercising. I was so excited that I couldn't wait to share the results with other people. I felt absolutely magnificent, as if I could spring like a majestic gazelle."

When Callan began teaching on her own, she instructed students privately in their homes. "I carried a metal pole with me from place to place to hang in doorways as a *barre*. We exercised on their living-room floors." Soon, she offered classes in her own studio apartment.

"It was a circus. I had a *barre* across my closet door. Students looked at my pitiful wardrobe while they exercised. I rearranged it every week so they wouldn't get bored at my interpretation of American clothes."

For the past seven years, Callan has been teaching in her penthouse that overlooks New York's East River.

There is no pulsating music, no shrill cadence called by an instructor. There is no grotesque machinery to make the place look like a modern-day torture chamber. Students, men and women of all ages, sizes, and shapes, work at their own speed under Callan's careful scrutiny. She moves about the room, attending to each individual's needs.

Callan's classes are a far cry from the usual fitness center environment: indoor-outdoor carpeting; wall-to-wall people blinding in fluorescent lighting; overly chlorinated pools; and a sea of humanity, everyone doing the same things at the same time, whether or not their bodies are capable of it.

A new student observed, "Coming to Callan's at seven o'clock in the morning is a terrific way to start the day. Someone wanders in at seven ten, someone else at seven twenty. Callan may be having breakfast or putting cream on her face, teaching while still in her nightgown. Despite this chaotic appearance, Callan has her hawkeye on everyone in the room. The way the mirrors are set up, she doesn't miss a trick.

"The sun comes through the greenhouse glass and literally bathes the room in warm light, exposing every roll and bump in your body. You see *exactly* what you look like on the beach and it scares the daylights out of you."

The natural light, reflected in the thirteen-foot mirrored walls, and the clear panorama of the city—the sky, rivers and skyscrapers—are magnificent inducements to exercise.

"One student told me that she had always thought her body was flawless . . . until she came here and saw it in bright light," Callan laughs. "I believe people need this kind of objectivity so that they will be able to *work* on their bodies."

There is a magnetic energy between Callan and her students. It's a powerful combination.

Callan Pinckney is a one-of-a-kind woman, and this is a one-of-a-kind book. Through it you will embark on a true adventure into body awareness . . . for obtaining your new, true shape of things to come.

—*Sallie Batson*

----------CHAPTER TWO----------

Excuses! Excuses! Excuses!

*I*f your personal exercise program never gets beyond the thinking stage, you must take a close look—a *very* close look—at what is keeping you from fitness. Read through this list of excuses and check off the ones you have used, and the ones you have thought of using, to explain why you are carrying around all that extra flab.

- ☐ I have big bones.
- ☐ It's my thyroid. My glands are really out of whack.
- ☐ I retain water.
- ☐ I might throw my back out.
- ☐ I hate to get all sweaty.
- ☐ My husband/wife/boyfriend/girlfriend likes me the way I am.
- ☐ I want to lose a little weight first. Then I'll start exercising.
- ☐ If I exercise now, all this fat will turn into muscle, and muscle is harder to lose than fat.
- ☐ I don't have time.
- ☐ My diet makes me too weak to exercise.
- ☐ If I had the kind of money he/she does, I'd look good too.
- ☐ Anybody can look great when they're sixteen.
- ☐ My whole family is big (fat).
- ☐ Exercise is boring.
- ☐ I've been sick.
- ☐ I have arthritis.

There are no excuses to keep anyone from tightening their thighs and lifting their behind for that wonderful, youthful feeling of childhood. Remember what that was like? If you can't, I'll remind you: When you walk, you feel as if puppet strings are pulling your buttocks into the air. If you never had that experience, it can be yours within hours, no matter your age, sex, or size. ▲

- ☐ I get enough exercise cleaning my house.
- ☐ I'm too tired to exercise when I come home from work.
- ☐ Once you've had a baby, your stomach goes to pot anyway.
- ☐ Saddle bags are a fact of life for women as we get older.
- ☐ I have to close this business deal first.
- ☐ Why should I lose? Men secretly like big women.
- ☐ I'm afraid I'll hurt myself.
- ☐ I just had my hair done.

Got the picture? I've heard them all, and so have you.

Quit whining. Put on some comfortable clothes and get to work on your body.

CHAPTER THREE

Chasing the Impossible Dream

*T*hings are not always what they seem, especially when you look at pictures of gorgeous bodies in magazines and, sadly, even in exercise books.

Every day, women around the world give up on their bodies because they can't transform themselves into the images of beauty created by the media. Who can compete with those incredibly young beauties in the fashion magazines? Real people like you and me could not possibly look like that!

No wonder we mere mortals suffer with low self-images. We buy every cosmetic on the market, try the latest hairstyles and fashions, use hip wraps and reducing creams, go on the latest diets, drink the right mineral waters, and we still fail to come close to Ideal Beauty.

My own lack of confidence in my body was due to conditioning. I had false expectations about how I should look. Despite years of compliments, I remained insecure about my appearance. New students, meeting me for the first time, often exclaimed, "You have the tightest, most beautiful body I've ever seen." I thought they were trying to flatter me so that I would go easy on them. It was impossible for me to consider. After all, I saw my body in the mirror every day. I knew what I looked like. How could they put *me* in the same league as those tall, exquisite young creatures in bathing suits cut up to their waists to show their perfect hips and legs?

I never suspected that the goddesses we see in the magazines don't always look that perfect either. I would have

Most weight loss by artistic means, be it airbrushing, cut-and-paste, or photography, is subtle: a bustline is raised, a hipline trimmed, a behind lifted and rounded, a waist cinched, and thighs slimmed and smoothed. These touches, as insignificant as they may seem, have monumental impact on the egos of unknowing women who think that what they see is real. To illustrate this point I have taken rather drastic steps, reducing a 230-pound woman to "normal" size. Were these photos used to advertise a diet or exercise plan, wouldn't you believe it worked? This is the only photograph in this book to receive any type of artistic editing. Every other body you see in the book or on the jacket is as it is in real life. ▶

This, and only this, photograph is airbrushed. ▲

sold my soul to have the body of one particular swimsuit model, until I saw her in person. I recognized her in a store where she was trying on high heels. As I watched her prance back and forth before the mirrors, I became more and more bewildered. She wore shorts. Her buttocks sagged and globs of cellulite sat on her hips. Her legs jiggled like tofu in a blender. I could not believe that the woman I had seen trying on shoes was the *real* person and the one in the magazines was the creation of a team of art directors, photographers, stylists, makeup artists, and airbrushers—The Army Corps of Image Engineers. You and I could look like the most beautiful women in the world too if we had this professional team to back us up.

Here's how they work:

The stylists—one for hair, one for makeup, and another for clothes—coif, curl, lift, paint, and primp you until there are no visible flaws.

You would then be directed to sit or stand about a perfectly appointed set, either in a photographer's studio or a real room, striking poses and moving in ways that show off your body to ultimate advantage.

Now, another sleight of hand begins. Lights are adjusted to create the desired (translate that "artificial") image, and a high-powered wind machine gives your hair and clothes that perfect billowy look. How many of us can lug around a four-foot fan to give us that perfect windblown look without a strand out of place?

Then, the photographer, using the appropriate cameras, lenses, films, filters, and angles, fires away, immortalizing your beauty in hundreds, if not thousands, of shots to obtain the *one* shining example of physical perfection.

If these techniques fail, have no fear: The cosmetic surgeons (known as the Art Department) can remedy anything else that may be considered wrong. They even correct any mistakes there might be in Mother Nature's handiwork. They operate on photographs, not living bodies.

Hips too wide? No problem. Able artists can use their scissors to cut off anything in the way, "amputating" bones if necessary, to give you a perfectly straight hipline.

Feet too big: again, no problem. They can chop off yours with scissors and glue on a prettier, younger, smoother, and yes, even smaller, pair in less time than it takes for you to slip into your stockings.

Flabby body but fabulous face? You can acquire a new figure, custom-made. Artists can superimpose your head and face onto the body of their choice. Or they can brush away any offending parts, such as thunder thighs, whale tails, droopy bosoms, tree-stump ankles, bulging bellies, and cellulite (or whatever you care to call those hideous ripply pockets of fat that so many women have). Gone, in an instant! Scissors, glue, and an airbrush machine—that's all an artist needs to create the most beautiful body in the world.

Airbrushing is one of the best kept secrets in this universe, outside of the advertising business. It is the final touch. This is a precision artistic technique, akin to spray painting, used to subtract or add parts of a picture. It can lighten or even remove shadows, iron out wrinkles in clothing *and* bodies, and take away any hair out of place. It can turn the *real* into the *perfectly unreal.*

No wonder we give up all hope of looking like the paper dolls in our favorite magazines. Our self-images are destroyed before we leave home!

Most women view their bodies as flawed. When someone comes to me for her first class, I ask her to stand in front of the mirrors and look objectively at her body. (I ask students not to wear tights—black tights hide multitudes of sins—or chic, belted leotards. I want them to wear something comfortable, yet revealing.) I ask her, "What would you like to change? What is it that you do not like about your body?" With nine out of ten of my students, the flaw they *think* they see is not a flaw at all.

Don't be tricked into thinking that everyone else you see is "perfect" and you are not. Work with what you have. There is always room for improvement. No one has a so-called perfect body.

I am writing about the methods of artistic deception because these techniques have damaged a lot of people. Every day I meet women and men who are depressed about their bodies. Many can't see how lovely, or potentially lovely, their bodies are.

It is harder for me to get a student to give up a negative self-image than it is for me to teach her how to exercise. I help my students to erase those false images that have been with them since their teens. I teach them how to see their bodies realistically and to stop chasing the impossible, retouched dream.

My student Page was an active, athletic teenager. However, when she went to college, she ate the typical cafeteria and junk foods that kept the average student alive. She ballooned before she took charge of her body and began a sensible routine of a nutritionally sound diet and my exercise program. Today her body is amazingly beautiful. It's better than airbrushing any day. ▲

CHAPTER FOUR

Portfolio of Proof

*T*he exercises you are about to learn produce fast results.

I could tell you that this is a complete, comprehensive program that will restore your body to its lithe, firm, young form and protect your back at the same time. And I could explain that if you follow the basic program outlined here, you can have a round, firm, peach-shaped behind, just like the little suntanned girl in the Coppertone suntan oil ads, in what seems like days. That is because an hour of these exercises equals approximately seven hours of conventional exercise and twenty hours of aerobic dancing, as far as firming the body and pulling it up is concerned.

Knowing your considerations, I have prepared a portfolio of pictures proving that these exercises work. By comparing the pictures of my students, you will be able to see for yourself that a flat, taut tummy and a high, round behind are possible for anyone who wants them.

To demonstrate the validity of my claim that these exercises work in a matter of hours, several of my students—all but one were beginners at the time—agreed to have their progress photographed for documentation. Some of these sequences were taken by a professional photographer. I took the others myself with a Polaroid camera. You will recognize the ones I took immediately! They were taken in the midst of dressing-room madness, hardly the best conditions for photography. On the pictures I took, you will see a line around the left-hand side of each body, thanks to less than perfect lighting. The darkroom technicians could have removed this photographic flaw, but I was committed to my promise that no pictures in this book would be altered.

For purposes of comparison, each student was photographed from the rear and in profile, immediately after class. The exact classes in each sequence are listed under each set of pictures. Samples of the progress made by participants in the project are included in this portfolio. One student, Jeanne,* was selected to show her hourly progress. Most of her photos are shown.

Joyce, my advanced student pictured here, became involved in the project when she told me that her body was "tight enough." She did not plan to continue classes because she did not see how her body could pull in any more than it already had. I picked up the challenge and said, "Let's take pictures and see." Joyce was surprised at the results. She had already pulled in dramatically and her continued progress was quite encouraging. I wasn't surprised. I see it happen every day. Unlike some other programs of exercise, this one continues to work as long as you do it.

Study the pictures. You can see a number of dramatic changes in each photo series. Hips become smaller and develop smoother lines. Behinds become higher, tighter, and rounder. Locate an identifying mark—a scar, birthmark, mole, stretchmarks, wrinkly fat deposits—and notice how they move higher and higher as the body becomes tighter.

If you see pouches of cellulite appear after you have worked to get your figure in shape, don't panic. The tightening from the exercises has only revealed what was there all along. My experience is that, if you change your diet, you can get rid of the unsightly, pebbly fat. For me, I eliminated coffee, red meats, dairy products, sugars, and processed foods from my diet. I ate a lot of vegetables and fish and drank at least eight glasses of water daily. I also took calcium supplements. My cellulite disappeared in six weeks.

Though their changes are not so radical, even men experience remarkable tightening and change. Women start out gooshier than men, so improvement is more visible from the start.

You can also see how students' postures improve. Remember what your mother said about standing up straight? Well, she had a point. Compare the first side views and subsequent side views of everyone in the portfolio. Notice how the bodies begin to change and how they become more and more erect. That's because the exercises tighten the hips and pull in the behind, which pulls in the inner thighs and, in turn, tips the pelvis up, which stretches the spine. The process reminds me of a Rube Goldberg contraption

*Names have been changed.

30

where you turn a tiny wheel to Point A, which sets off a sequence of reactions to make the cage fall on the mouse at Point Z.

The entire figure-shaping process is accomplished automatically—the way Nature intended. However, for most of us, Nature needs a boost. That's where these exercises come in. See for yourself how well they work.

LUCY
Age: 40

After 1st Class

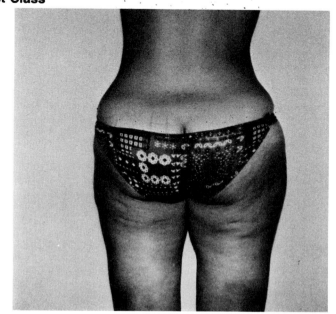

After 4th Class

GERTRUDE
Age: 32

After 1st Class

After 3rd Class

After 4th Class

After 5th Class

MARCIE
Age: 37

After 1st Class

After 7th Class

CHRISTINE
Age: 27

After 1st Class

After 5th Class

MARK
Age: 27

After 1st Class

After 4th Class

JOYCE
Age: 28

After 14th Class

After 24th Class

CHARLES
Age: 41

After 2nd Class

After 9th Class

JEANNE
Age: 32

After 1st Class

After 2nd Class

After 4th Class

After 6th Class

After 7th Class

After 10th Class

After 11th Class

After 13th Class

After 14th Class

After 15th Class

After 16th Class

After 17th Class

After 18th Class

After 19th Class

JEANNE
Age: 32

After 1st Class

After 19th Class

──────── **CHAPTER FIVE** ────────

What Makes These Exercises Special?

*E*xercising should not be a second job with no salary, a chore with no reward. Time is money. Energy is precious. Why squander them on something futile?

I have taught exercise to thousands of people, ranging in age from eight to eighty-plus, during the past twelve years, with magnificent, rapid success. The movements I teach produce results in *hours,* not days, weeks, or months. The term "year" is unheard of when discussing getting in shape by this plan.

My impatience with the unnecessary effort and time demanded by conventional figure-trimming programs—aerobic dance, weights and exercise machines, calisthenics and ordinary isometrics included—prompted me to write this book. Life is too short to spend in a gym.

My students don't spend an hour a day working out. Who has that kind of time? Exercising is boring, boring, boring! Why be bored when you can get on with life? Spend your time on something that works. After the first hour of class, my students *feel* a difference in their bodies; after the second, most actually *see* it.

It's quite an adventure. In no time at all you will have restored your body to its lithe, firm, young form without injury—especially to your back—and without going to a gym or investing in expensive equipment.

If you're interested in rejuvenating your body and reclaiming your right to have a fantastic figure, it's not too late to start, no matter your age, sex, or physical condition. When I first began exercising, I felt like I had a toothache all over

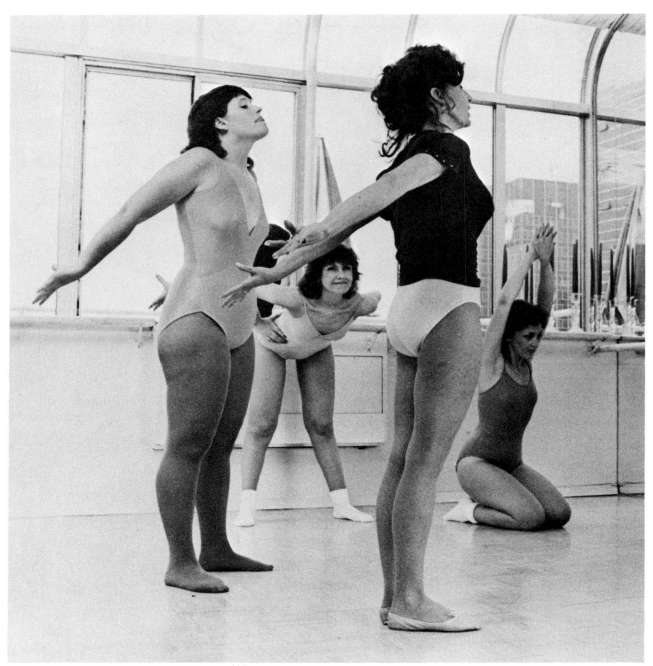

When you start exercising, do the complete program, from warm-up to inner thigh squeeze. In most classes, someone may be starting the warm-ups while another student may be working on her hips and behind, and another, her pelvis. Exercising is a very personal experience. Make the time you spend working on your body work for you. ▲

my body. Dancing, and most other activities I enjoyed, were out of the question because of my back pain and overall lack of muscle tone. Now look at me. You too can have the body you deserve if you're willing to work for it.

First, throw away your scales, or at least stash them in a closet where you won't be tempted to weigh every time you walk past them. Your body will quickly begin to go through some rather impressive changes. If you weigh yourself to check your daily progress, you may be in for quite a shock. The scale will not reflect your success as truthfully as your mirror and your clothes.

The important thing is how your body responds to the care it gets from your exercising. Exercise, in general, promises strength, endurance, and flexibility. This program has nine additional benefits:

- Coordination
- Balance
- Comprehensive body awareness
- Body control
- Discipline
- Speed
- Physical and mental relaxation
- Builds stamina
- Decreases appetite

When you start doing these exercises, you will no doubt discover more important pluses of your own. As you start to pull in, you will experience some surprising changes. For one, you may even show a weight *gain* of up to six or seven pounds. The trauma of putting on poundage could be so startling that it might throw you off your program. It is not uncommon for students to gain pounds, according to the scale, while dropping two or even three dress sizes. Every pound you lose looks like two.

There is a very rational explanation to this rather irrational occurrence. There is less muscle than flab to a pound. (Remember your high school science: A pound of feathers and a pound of steel weigh the same, but the pound of feathers takes up more room than the pound of steel because of the *volume* of feathers needed to make up that pound.)

Don't be frightened by the wonderful changes taking place within your body. These initial fluctuations are immaterial when you consider how beautiful your body is becoming.

WHAT MY STUDENTS AND I
WEAR TO EXERCISE

An exercise session is *not* a fashion show. I personally don't care what anyone wears, as long as they are comfortable. You can wear a burlap bag, as long as your body is not restricted by what you have on.

When the pictures were being taken for this book, some of my students had to buy leotards or borrow from friends, because most of them do not wear them in class. Their usual garb is decidedly less photogenic: gym shorts and torn T-shirts, jogging suits, loose sweatshirts over dance shorts. Instead of leg warmers, most wear crew socks. We're a motley crew!

No one would have minded being photographed in their ordinary class clothes, but aesthetic wisdom prevailed. It was important to show the precise movements of the exercises as clearly as possible. That would have been impossible if everyone wore baggy warm-up suits.

Students of all sizes and shapes demonstrate the exercises and are in the group pictures. Most are new students.

Another reason I advise my students not to bother with dancewear for exercise is that people tend to spend too much time comparing what they have on with the latest status leotard-and-tights look.

Work on your body, not on your wardrobe of exercise clothes. Save your money for a few weeks and splurge on a gorgeous dress or a beautifully fitted pair of pants! Save your fashion energy for when you get your body looking beautiful, are going out with the man of your dreams, and you want to look and feel like a queen!

Tights are not essential to proper exercise either. In fact they can be a detriment to the full benefits of your program. Tights are appropriately named, indeed, especially those of Lycra and spandex, which are like leg girdles. They press your leg muscles and lessen the contractions of the exercises. They also inhibit circulation while hiding what you should be seeing.

Belted exercise uniforms are more fashionable than functional. I have seen women cinch their belts so tightly that their waists look gorgeous, but they can hardly breathe properly, much less bend over. The purpose of exercise is to make your waist smaller. The purpose of wearing a belted exercise costume is to make it *look* smaller.

WHAT, NO SOUNDS OF MUSIC?

Music may be exciting or soothing, but I prefer to teach without this distraction. The music gets between you and your mastery of your body.

When learning these movements, pay attention to your movements. If you are playing music with a driving beat, you instinctively move your body in time. Therefore, you forfeit control of the exercises.

Until you have perfected the techniques of these exercises, silence is golden indeed.

A WORD ABOUT TEMPERATURES

Leave your sweaty gym mentality with your scales when you begin this program! You won't need it to shape up.

Unless the temperature and the humidity are hideously high, I do not turn on the air-conditioners in my studio. I have the windows open and I use a ceiling fan that cools the air without stirring up a draft.

Exercising in an air-conditioned room can cause you to get a chill and, as a result, experience painful muscle cramps. Stay out of drafts, regardless of how hot you get. Dry off and get out of your exercise clothes before you become chilled and your muscles cramp.

The perspiration generated by exercise is one way the body regulates its temperature. It has very little to do with long-term weight loss. The weight loss by heavy perspiration is only temporary because it is, in truth, water loss.

Often my students sip water in between sets of exercises because they feel thirsty. Fruit juices and soft drinks, however, defeat the purpose of exercise. Juices and sodas are usually too sweet to quench your thirst. (Juices are also higher in calories than fruits.)

WHERE SHOULD YOU EXERCISE?

These exercises can be done anywhere, anytime. As long as you are comfortable.

Ideally, you should have a mirror—a big one—so that you can see how your body is positioned. Don't be intimidated. I lived in my mirrored apartment for a year before I really looked at myself. I was very conscious of avoiding my reflection. I was afraid that my body wouldn't look as youthful and tight as I wanted. One day I was exercising alone. It was summer. The sun was streaming through the greenhouse walls, bathing my body in a brutal light. I could see every lump and bump . . . only there weren't any. At last I felt wonderful about my body.

While you don't need any special equipment to do these exercises properly, you will need a secure *barre* for some of the exercises you do to trim and firm your legs and, especially, for working on your behind and hips. Rather than install rigging as I have done in my studio, use your imagination—a kitchen counter, a strong table, the back of your couch, or even your bureau top.

Find something other than a towel rack for support. Even the ones that are cemented in tile to the walls of your bathroom are too insecure to bear more weight than a couple of wet towels. The type that is screwed into the wall is even more dangerous, especially since you may be tempted to hold on for dear life until you build up your strength enough to use the *barre*—or whatever substitute you adopt—for balance.

Anyone can do these exercises. Even people who consider themselves Super Klutzes—they can't walk and talk at the same time—gain control of their bodies. Every person I have taught, regardless of his or her age or condition, who had the determination to have a strong, fit, and beautiful body, now has it.

The complete program, as it is constructed, can be done in less than an hour, once you have gained enough strength to do the exercises. This can be divided to fit your day's schedule. Break it up so that it suits you.

You will want to do the One-Hour Program twice a week at first. Once you have your figure the way you want it, you may adopt the 15-Minute Maintenance Plan as your primary exercise routine, doing the complete workout once a week . . . or when it's time to whip your body back into shape—after the holidays, for example.

Once you experience the deep contractions of these innovative exercises and see how quickly your body pulls in, you will *make* time for yourself. These exercises will become the highlight of your day.

CHAPTER SIX

The One-Hour Program

You are now ready to give yourself one of the most wonderful gifts in the world: a fabulous, tight, *fit* figure. It is only hours away if you follow the plan detailed in the pages ahead.

The One-Hour Program I teach is explained in detail in the following chapters in such a way that you will be able to follow the instructions and photographs movement by movement. These are not your ordinary exercises, therefore I have been very explicit, almost repetitious, in explaining how every exercise should be done. Since I won't be there to demonstrate and to position your body before you start, I have taken every care that you will know what to do.

Each set of exercises is designed to work on a specific part of the body. In each chapter you will see precisely how to execute the delicate movements and deep contractions that give the exercises their power, and you will see the exact parts of your body that will benefit from each section.

The people demonstrating the program had been to fewer than four classes at the time we took their photos. They are doing the exercises as best as their bodies will allow—or, I should say, *allowed*—when the pictures were taken.

That is all I ask of anyone who does this program. Do what you can. As you become stronger, you will be able to do more and more with ease. You will feel your muscles contract more deeply and you will stretch more fully when your body is ready.

Do not force your body to do anything it is not prepared to

Classes are a free-for-all at my studio. Everyone works at their own pace and sees and feels results in hours, not weeks or months or more. There is no music, no dance routine and no machine and weight program—just a program of very personal, very practical body movements. ▲

do. If instructions say "Put your foot on the *barre*" and you cannot lift your leg all the way up to the kitchen counter that you are using as your exercise *barre,* don't even attempt it. Rest your foot on a sturdy, low chair. Once your hamstrings and spine are stretched and your entire body is ready for you to raise your leg as high as that counter, you will be able to accomplish it with graceful ease.

Take frequent breathers at first. If you feel a burning sensation in muscles after you have done twenty-five or thirty repetitions when instructions say you are to do one hundred, stop what you are doing and shift your position. This may mean your muscles aren't strong enough yet. Try working on the opposite side, so that your muscles can rest. Or, it may mean that you need to lie down flat and rest for a few minutes.

When you stop an exercise, rest and then start over again *from the original starting position.* Repeat it step by step. In this way, you will be certain that your body is properly positioned for safety and the success of the exercise.

I do not teach any special breathing technique because I have found that people pay so much attention to their breathing that they forget to exercise. Just remember to breathe naturally. If you hold your breath you are only denying your body the oxygen it must have to cleanse the blood and nourish your muscles. Without it you won't have the stamina you deserve.

I have two very specific words of warning. Please take them to heart.

To Pregnant Women: Under no circumstances should any woman in the first trimester of pregnancy do the stomach exercises unless her doctor has actually gotten down on the floor and done them to feel how deep the contractions are. Don't just show your Ob-Gyn the book. The exercises appear to be very easy, but looks, in this case, are terribly deceiving.

This is not to say that expectant mothers cannot do the program. I will take a woman after her fourth month if she will agree to make an appointment for the two of us to show the exercises to her gynecologist or obstetrician. I have the doctor get down and do them.

Mothers who have been in the program before they became pregnant or began it after their fourth month tell me that they had incredibly easy deliveries and amazing recovery rates.

To Everyone: I ask you to have your doctor check you over before you begin this, or any other, physical fitness regimen. We have all heard this warning before and all of us have gone ahead and exercised without benefit of a checkup. A lot of people have been severely injured. Because of the nature of these exercises, I ask that this time you pay attention; get your doctor's go-ahead. I have had no known injuries as a result of these exercises in the twelve years I have been teaching, but I won't be there to supervise you.

Now, we are ready to begin.

You will probably notice that your body is shifting after your second hour if you follow the program exactly, from warm-up to inner thigh squeeze, with everything in between, each time you exercise.

To say it another way: If you want with all your heart to get rid of your thunder thighs and think you can do *only* the exercises for the behind and hips and have your dream come true, you are only fooling yourself.

Follow the program as it is written. That works.

If you have weak stomach muscles, your stomach may appear larger at first, even though your waist is already smaller. You are working on your upper stomach muscles first. Also your hips are pulling in and your behind is rising. Keep working. All of a sudden your abdominal muscles will catch up with the rest of your newly-firm body and be beautifully flat.

As your hips and behind pull in and up, you may notice a lump of flesh just below your waist in the back, where you feel when you put your hands on your hips. Don't get hysterical like I did. As everything tightens, all that gooshy mass on your hips is being lifted and tightened to be a high, round, firm behind! Keep at it.

Here are more surprises that you may have ahead:

- One morning you will notice in the mirror that your neck is longer and narrower.
- As if by magic, your inner thighs will look smooth and part of your legs, not something mushy and separate.
- Your legs will look longer and leaner and you will feel as though you have the spring of a gazelle.
- One night you will roll over in bed and feel as if your cat had left a toy under the covers and it is poking into your

hip. It's your hipbone. Your stomach has become so tight and flat that your hipbones show.

You are truly able to resculpt your body into an image of beauty. It won't be a breeze, but it will be fast.

Laugh at yourself if your body won't cooperate. Talk to your muscles, caress them, cajole them, tease them, and soon you will be able to get them to do anything you ask. Each hour of exercise you do, your body becomes stronger and firmer . . . and lovelier.

It's so exciting.

One Final Word: Please read the instructions for each exercise thoroughly before beginning the movements.

CHAPTER SEVEN

Warming Up

*D*on't think you can let yourself off easy if you skip over these warm-ups and right into the real body work. If you do, you are asking for trouble.

Contrary to the casual-sounding name, warm-ups are not "nonexercises" that are done before you do an exercise program. Quite literally, warming up means that you warm up your muscles. You elevate your body temperature and increase cardiovascular activity to send blood and oxygen throughout your body.

Many years ago, I asked doctors and therapists what should be done in a warm-up and could not get a straight answer. So I tried my own experiment. For two weeks I had one particular class do only stretches to "warm up," while the rest of my classes did my regular program of warm-up exercises and stretches. The test class did not perform well at all. I concluded that their muscles were stretched but they certainly weren't warmed up.

Dancers are known to spend forty-five minutes or more limbering up before a performance. One high kick could tear an unprepared hamstring to shreds. A muscle spasm might cause a fall that could end a career.

This heightened activity prepares the muscles for the more strenuous, demanding activity ahead. Muscles are gently stretched and flexed, joints are put through their range of motion, all to protect the body from injury. Because you have given your body a taste of the delicious results of exercise, you will be able to work safely and completely on your entire body.

My classes are informal, intimate. It is a safe, comfortable environment for my students to work on their bodies. Classes small—seven students, tops—and there's nothing regimented to force anyone to do something they aren't ready for. You could easily create the same secure intimacy in your home, or at the home of a friend, and start your own exercise group. There is something about having a specific time and place, where you regularly join the same group of friends, that makes starting an exercise program fun. ▲

Each of these gentle, seemingly simple warm-ups is perfect preparation for the deep contractions and the precise, accurate movements inherent in the remainder of this one-hour program.

Pat, who is demonstrating this part of the program, had completed three classes at the time of the photography session. She is in her mid-fifties, a highly-motivated professional woman who is also the mother of teenagers.

WARM-UP #1 *Stretch your spine by hanging. Let your body drip to the floor like melting wax. If you don't have access to a ladder, as I have in my studio, or a chinning bar, grasp the top of a sturdy door braced open against a wall and covered with a towel to protect your hands. If you use a door, you will have to face it in order to hold on. Otherwise, reach around the bar and hold as Pat is doing. Don't be afraid that you will fall, or you will make the mistake of tensing your entire body. That defeats the purpose of the stretch. Hold as long as you can—even if only for a second—with your feet off the floor. If you're too tall, bend your knees. Point your toes if you can. Feel your body stretch and lengthen. When I started hanging, I could only hold for a fast count of 5. Now, my wrists and arms are so strong, I can hang for a slow count of 75 or more. If you are lucky enough to live near a playground or schoolyard, you can hang from the swings or jungle gym. ▶*

WARM-UP #2 *Stand erect with your feet about a foot apart—but never more than 15 inches—and raise your chest upward. Lift both arms over your head, reaching high. Keep reaching. You want to stretch your stomach, making you feel as if your torso is 2 inches longer than it really is.*

Bend your knees, keeping your feet flat on the floor. Continue stretching upward. Bend your upper body forward, arms out, as though reaching for something in front of you. Continue to stretch your torso outward. Still bending your knees and leaning forward, bring your arms to your sides, even with your calves. ▲

Continue to raise your arms up behind your body, stretching your neck out as you do this. Keep knees relaxed and body bent over. Do not arch your back. Keep shoulders relaxed and rounded. Complete this exercise by reversing the movements to the starting position. Do 5, returning the arms to the initial stretching position between each combination. ▼

FOR TIGHTENING THE UNDERARMS *This is the* only *underarm exercise you need to do. Standing erect, as for the initial warm-up, reach arms outward to the sides at shoulder level and roll them forward so that the palms face upward. The more you turn your arms so that your palms are pointing to the sky, the more you will feel. Gently take your arms behind you, as if you were trying to make your shoulder blades meet. Move only a half inch at a time back and forth behind you. Do not jerk. Hold your head and shoulders back. Tighten your behind and hold your stomach in as you tip your pelvis upward. Relax your legs. Do 100, trying to touch thumbs. Keep your arms turned over behind your back and keep your thumbs up. The higher you can hold your arms straight the more you will feel the muscle working. Do not bend your elbows. Done properly, this exercise tightens your underarms and pectoral muscles, which raises the bustline and loosens tension in the muscles between your shoulder blades and neck.* ▼

WAIST STRETCH *Stand with feet about a foot apart and arms at your sides. Raise your right arm high over your head and place your left hand on the outside of your left leg. Stretch your right arm and the right side of your body upward, straightening your right elbow. Reach your right arm about 2 inches higher than you think you can. Do not arch your back. Tighten your behind and tip your pelvis upward. Hold position.* ▲

Stretch your right arm up and over to the left side, bending your left elbow as you lean. Keep reaching over your head with your right arm, keeping it straight to stretch your underarm and the back of your shoulders. Reach over your head as though you are trying

to touch something on a table at your left side with your right hand. Soon you will be stretching so far that you will be reaching for something on the floor. Keep your pelvis tilted forward and your behind tucked and tight at all times to stretch the spine. From that point, reach over a half inch more, gently moving up and down, a half inch each way, 100 times. Do not bounce or throw your hip out to the side. Hips and pelvis never leave their starting positions. Do not allow your left elbow to slip to the back or to the front. To change sides, gently reach forward with your right arm, bending your body from the waist to the front. Keep your left hand on your left leg and turn your entire upper body to the right, gently returning to a standing position. Put your right hand on your right leg and raise your left arm high over your head. Proceed from there, repeating 100 times in each direction. Done properly, this waist stretch will stretch your underarms, the backs of your shoulders, and your waist and spine. It's essential to learn to do this properly because as your hips become smaller, you have to work harder to keep your waist looking small. ▲

HAMSTRING STRETCH *This is a classic, though controversial, stretching exercise. Some experts advise people with back trouble to avoid it, and others recommend it. I, with my history of back problems, do it with no difficulty. Similarly, my students who have back problems report that their backs feel wonderful once they learn it correctly. From a standing position—the basic starting position—bend forward from the waist with your arms out in front of you. Keep knees bent. Gently touch your palms to the floor, if you can. Pat could not do this at first. However, after only three classes, she was able to. Never lock your knees. If you are not stretched enough to touch the floor with ease, bend your knees, as Pat is doing in the pictures. Although she was already able to straighten her legs while touching the floor, I felt it essential to show you how beginners start. All I ask is that you do what you can.* ▲

Gently grasp the insides of your legs, as low as you can, with your hands. Keep your body relaxed, shoulders rounded, and head tucked under. Bend your elbows outward to stretch between your shoulder blades. Gently move your torso a half inch, or as close to that as you can, between your legs. Do not bounce. Relax your neck. Do 20. ▲

Do not *come back up. Move your left hand behind the left calf and bring your right arm over, clasping your left leg just below your left hand, above your left ankle. Bend your elbows out like a duck's wings. Tuck your head between your*

left leg and right arm, as though you were trying to look behind you. Stretch as far as you can without straining, then relax. Count to 20. Without standing up, change to your right side, *gently and slowly moving to that side, and repeat for 20 counts. Return both hands to the floor in front of you without forcing and arch your back upward like a cat, slowly straightening one vertebra at a time, until you are standing erect. This hamstring stretch also gives your calves, waist, lower back, and the muscles between your shoulder blades a good workout. Remember: Practice keeping your knees relaxed, not locked, throughout the exercise or you are inviting damage to your knee-joint complexes. The more stretched your hamstrings become, the more you will be able to straighten your legs.* ▲

NECK EXERCISE #1 *From the initial stance, slowly lower your head, chin to chest. Relax your shoulders. Tighten your behind and tip your pelvis upward. Tighten your stomach as you stretch your neck upward.* ▶

Slowly and smoothly roll your head to one side, lifting your chin as far as you can toward the ceiling. Keep your shoulders relaxed and your behind tight. Remember to make all movements extremely gently. Your neck is a delicate construction of bone and tissue that can be damaged by hard or jerky movements. Let your shoulders drop toward the floor. This is a common mistake— tensing the shoulders and holding them up. Still moving slowly and gently, roll your head to the opposite side, lifting your chin as far as you can to that side. Do 5 in each direction. ▶

NECK EXERCISE #2 *As in the preceding exercise, this is for pure relaxation while loosening the neck and shoulders. Stand straight, tummy tight and behind and pelvis tipped forward and up. Relax your shoulders and arms and stretch your body upward. Hold your head and neck as high as you can. Then, as slowly as you can, move your head to one side without moving your body or shoulders. Pretend you are trying to look behind you without moving anything but your head. Hold for a slow count of 5 and gently move your head to the other direction. Do 5 in each direction.* ▲

CHAPTER EIGHT

For the Stomach

At first glance, these look like many other stomach exercises you have seen in magazines and books. However, you will find that they are very different indeed.

They are not sit-ups, nor are they backward rolls. They are precise, concentrated movements that contract and release the entire network of muscles that lace across the stomach from breast to pubis. The effect is so powerful that it benefits the body all the way to the chin in sixteen very specific ways. The following exercises:

- Tighten all four sections of the abdominal muscles, from breastbone to crotch.
- Release tension in the back of the neck.
- Lengthen the neck.
- Release tension across the shoulder blades.
- Expand breathing capacity by expanding the chest.
- Lift the breasts by working the pectoral muscles.
- Eliminate double chins.
- Release tension and stretch the *entire* back, including the sacrum.
- Usually relieve menstrual cramping for most women who experience this.
- Benefit the cardiovascular system.
- Usually regulate bowel movements for most people with irregularity and diarrhea.
- Increase body awareness.
- Teach coordination.
- Enable you to relax.
- Decrease appetite.
- Increase your sexual drive—like it or not!

These powerful exercises are not simple to do. Often, I pass among my students and lend a hand where I am needed, or correct students who are not executing the movements properly or safely. It is important that you move your head, shoulders, and arms as one unit, without rocking your body back and forth. ▲

Each one of these exercises does all this. As with all the exercises you will see here, they build stamina, endurance, and strength.

What makes them so special is that *you* have complete control over each movement. Regardless of the basic starting position, you determine when and how much you move. You control the movement, rather than letting the movement control you.

For most of us, once we reach a certain point in a backward roll, we no longer have control over how fast we roll our bodies back. Gravity takes over. When we do a series of sit-ups, we begin by pulling upright and easing down to the floor, never realizing that a sit-up involves, conservatively, 80 to 85 percent of the back muscles. Once we gather momentum, we yank our torsos to a sitting position and collapse back to the floor.

With this series, you won't find your body or even gravity taking over the activity. Once you have learned to position your body and move properly, you will be able to feel every contraction and every release of every muscle involved, regardless of how deep. This is because you learn to isolate your muscles and move only certain groups to achieve specific results.

The more you control your muscles, the more you will be able to tighten and trim your stomach. The abdominal muscles will form a taut resilient girdle that holds you flat and young-looking regardless of your age or sex. Even women who have had children experience a tightening that they won't get from aerobic dancing or yoga.

I know of no other exercise program that gives contractions as deep and powerful as these. That is why they work so well. I have had students who were extremely overweight when they started classes. Every one of them who stuck with me found positive, dramatic results from following these essential stomach exercises. Others who, once they were past their first trimesters, exercised through their pregnancies, felt fabulous for it. Every one of them reported easy deliveries and each was able to get her firm figure back much faster than her friends who did other exercises.

These exercises may feel a bit unusual at first. You may not feel the contractions in your stomach muscles at all because you are concentrating on the tension—the ache—in the back of your neck. Unless you are *really* tense, this disappears after your first hour; whatever tightness you may feel in the sides of your neck, gone after the second. By your third hour, you should feel no pain in any part of your neck. Then you will really get a sense of how strong the contractions in your stomach are.

Tension in the neck and upper body may also be felt between or across the shoulder blades after the first few hours. As you exercise, this tension is released and you acquire full movement in your shoulders and upper torso. (If this continues past the fourth hour, your body might be telling you to see your doctor about possible disc problems.)

The deeper the muscles work, the less you will be able to do. When your muscles become stronger at a deeper level, the more repetitions you will be able to do. When one layer of muscles have been completely worked, the layer below will take over.

If you have weak stomach muscles, the contractions will begin under your bustline. The stronger, more relaxed these muscles are, the higher you will be able to pull your shoulders and upper body, which will result in deeper, lower contractions of the stomach and abdomen.

I cannot remind you enough: Each movement you make is gentle, small. Move no more than half an inch in either direction where movement is called for. Your head, shoulders, and upper torso are a unit. Do not rock your body back and forth or tighten your behind. These are not exercises to be done with your head. Relax. You may find this difficult at first, but practice keeping your legs loosened and relaxed.

As your hips and thighs tighten and your upper stomach muscles become firm and flat, your lower abdomen may appear to be puffier than when you started. This is an illusion. After very few sessions, you will find that the muscles flatten right across your tummy and your hipbones will show.

Don't worry about your breathing. Exhale as you pull yourself up; otherwise, breathe naturally.

I start students out with one hundred of each exercise. As each section of muscle is strengthened, you may feel that you are starting all over again and can only do a fourth of what you did the class before, because your muscles are working more deeply. You have progressed to another level. Keep going. Soon you will be able to do the full number again.

Twenty-two-year-old Lisa is a transplanted Texan who came to New York to expand her career as an actress. She had had only three classes when these pictures were taken. **Note:** Common mistakes at first are bouncing your head, only moving your arms, rocking your body back and forth, holding your breath, not relaxing your body, and tightening your behind.

For the Stomach

FOR THE STOMACH #1 *Lie on the floor, relaxing your entire body, with your arms at your sides and your knees up. Feet should be 3 to 5 inches apart. Push the small of your back into the floor.* ◄

With your head and shoulders still on the floor, firmly grab hold of your inner thighs and raise your elbows up and out to each side to stretch between shoulder blades. Don't be gentle—grab. ►

71

Pulling on your inner thighs, pull your head and shoulders off the floor, rounding upward from under the bust. The small of your back should still be pushed into the floor. ▲

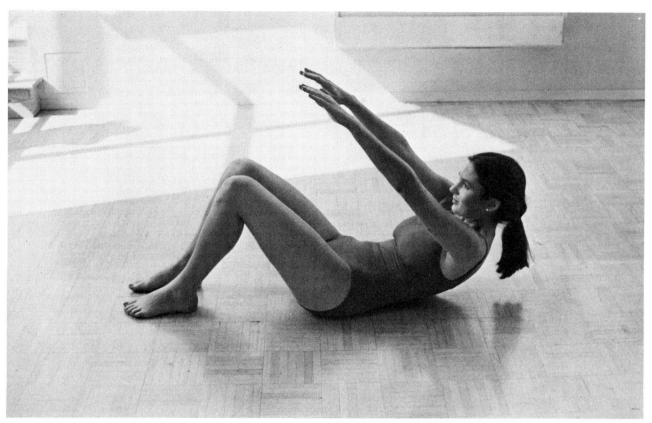

Release hands from inner thighs and raise arms parallel with your thighs and knees. Do not let your head and shoulders fall back to the floor. From that position, lift your arms, shoulders, and head as one unit a half inch further from the floor. Only the top of your body moves. Move slowly back a half inch, again using only the top part of your body. Move upper torso back and forth, in triple slow motion, a half inch in each direction; do this 2 more times than you think you can. Then rest. Aim for 75 at your first class, but stop when you feel you must. When you feel that you can do no more, gently let your body roll down to the floor, vertebra by vertebra, and take a breather. Then, repeating each step from the beginning, come back up and continue. Do not rock back and forth. Keep behind still. If you feel this in the back of your neck at first, this is natural. You are beginning to loosen up stored tension. If it really hurts, clasp your hands behind your head, just above your neck, and let your head rest in the palms of your hands. Take your elbows out to the sides as far as you can. ▲

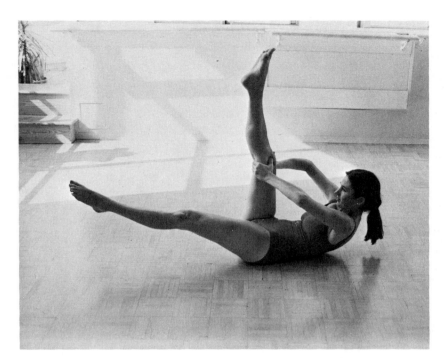

FOR THE STOMACH #2 *Lie on your back on the floor, both legs straight and together. From that position, raise the right leg toward the ceiling and lift left leg a foot off the floor. Grab the back of your right knee with both hands, round your elbows outward and up toward the ceiling, and pull your head and shoulders up toward your knee as high as you can. Keep the small of your back pressed into the floor. Do not point your toes or tighten legs at first. Relax. Think of them as feathers.* ◄

When you feel you can't bring your head and shoulders any higher, let go of your raised knee and stretch arms toward your right foot. Move your upper torso back and forth a half inch in triple slow motion. Do 100 times with each leg raised, taking breathers when necessary. If you have average stomach muscles, you will only be able to move up and down a half inch. Keep your back pressed into the floor. The important thing about this exercise is not to see how high you can move your chest but how rounded you can curl your upper body. If you feel your lower back working for this exercise, either rest your left leg on the floor or put your left foot on the floor and bend your knee upward. Keep your raised leg high to discourage your lower back muscles from assisting your abdominals. When your stomach muscles are strong enough, you can lower your legs as low as you wish. If you feel a burning sensation between your shoulder blades, nine times out of ten it simply means that your muscles are tight and are beginning to loosen up. ▲

Note: When you are lying on your back, always bend your knees and then straighten your legs upward; otherwise, you will exert pressure on your lower back.

FOR THE STOMACH #3 *Lie on the floor with both legs in the air. Grab the outer thighs with your hands and, rounding your shoulders and elbows out, pull your head and shoulders up toward your knees. Pull as high as you can, with your lower back pushed into the floor.* ▶

Let go of your legs and stretch hands and arms toward your toes. Do not let your head and shoulders fall back to the floor. Gently lift the top of your body up and down a half inch to an inch for a count of 100. Again, keep your legs relaxed. If you have weak legs, you can bend your knees. At first, you will probably not be able to let your legs go down as far as Lisa can. Your legs will be up higher. ◀

For People Who Find It Difficult to Keep Their Legs Up *Rest your feet on a wall, as shown, again pulling yourself up on your outer thighs. Let go and stretch your hands toward your feet. Gently move up and down. Keep your knees bent to avoid pressure on your legs. When you are strong enough to take your legs off the wall, they should feel like feathers.* ▶

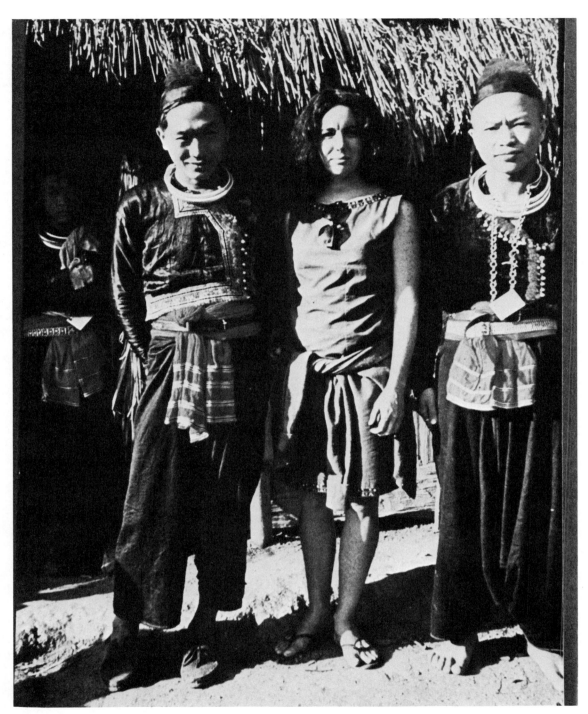

My stomach was distended from malnutrition and, though I weighed only about 80 pounds, I was so bloated that I looked larger than I am now. (I wore a Size 6 dress then. Today, I fluctuate between 100 and 105 pounds, but my body is so tight I wear a Size 2.) My mother showed this photo, taken among a Laotian mountain tribe, for several months before she recognized me by the crease in my brow. My body had deteriorated so much that I had no muscle tone and no strength. Still in my twenties, I looked and felt 120! ▲

CHAPTER NINE

For the Legs

I tell my students that we all can have long, thin, tight-looking legs like Cyd Charisse. It's all in the exercises we do.

The legs are the one part of a woman's body that can be overdeveloped in a very short time. All it takes is certain body movements—too much contraction, the use of weights, even the wrong exercises. In a matter of days, thighs and calves can become hard and mannishly muscular. Or, they can become long looking and thin.

I know this firsthand. A nurse asked if she might use two-and-a-half-pound ankle weights so that the exercises for the hips and behind might work faster. Against my better judgment, I decided to give them a try. We both questioned how this might affect the knees and hip joints, but I went ahead with the experiment. In a total of thirty minutes of exercise over a three-day period, my knees became terribly swollen and painful. My right hip hurt so much that I had to use a hot, moist heating pad to relieve the ache. If that wasn't bad enough, varicose veins appeared behind my knees and on the sides. I had aggravated my knee problems, which I had not experienced in years. My knees were so distorted, and legs larger, from this small amount of weight work, that twice I had to cancel photography sessions for this book. I feared that my knees might never return to their better shape.

Needless to say, my students who witnessed this are nervous about weights now—especially when they saw how bad my knees looked! It took at least a month for all the swelling to go down.

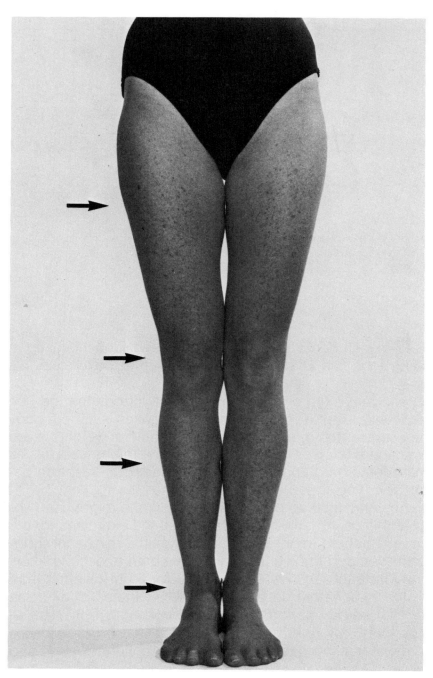

When I was a child, I saw a large photograph in Life magazine of what was supposed to be "The Perfect Legs." Four 50-cent pieces were placed between the model's legs at the four places where a woman's legs should touch: thighs, knees, calves, and ankles. I never forgot that image and have strived to achieve that look through the years. Now, at age forty-five, I can honestly say that I have not merely acquired the look in the magazine, I have surpassed it. Through the proper stretching and contractions, I have rid myself of the knotty calf muscles that so many ballet dancers get. ▲

A man, on the other hand, could double the work that I did with weights, and his legs would generally look better for doing it.

The exercises I teach do not build bulk or increase your thighs and cause hamstring bulge. They do just enough to create a light, firm, long look without hulking, protruding muscles. We short women must be especially careful about becoming too muscular because, on us, bulky muscles make our legs look wide and shorter than they already are. As a result, our *bodies* look stubby and ugly.

To some extent, these leg exercises come from my ballet training—*pliés* and *barre* work, in particular—yet they are designed to care for the delicate mechanisms of the knees, hips, and ankles.

I must caution anyone who has had knee problems to see their doctor before attempting these, or any other, exercises that use the legs. Out of hundreds of students who have come to me with bad knees, all but one experienced relief. The one who did not get noticeably better did admit that although she had not experienced any *improvement* while doing the exercises, she had not gotten any worse. She then admitted that when she stopped doing the exercises altogether, her pain increased.

I can't remind you enough: Do what you can. Don't force your leg higher than it can easily reach. *Never* jerk your body. Abrupt movement is a primary cause of injury, no matter what kind of exercise you do. Don't expect to move and look like a prima ballerina—or even like Katie, my student who is demonstrating these exercises for you—the first time you try them. At first, you will find it impossible to keep your shoulders erect and your behind tight at the same time. You may also feel like you are clinging to the *barre* for dear life. Don't worry. As you become stronger, all this will become much easier.

Katie, a thirty-year-old mother with a small child, had completed three classes at the time of our pictures. She did the exercises as well as her body allowed at that time.

Note: I teach the first two exercises for the legs with the heels together, balancing on the balls of the feet. Katie, however, found it more comfortable to do them with her heels slightly apart. I have found that with the heels together you get more relief from pressure on the knees, since the body's weight is centered over the heels instead of through the knees. Also, with heels together, the inner thighs work more, taking pressure off the knees. At first, if you are un-

79

comfortable, like Katie, in that position, you may feel free to take them apart to achieve a balanced stance. The exercises will still work.

FOR THE LEGS #1 *Gently clasp the back of a sturdy chair or sofa, or even the kitchen counter, with both hands at shoulder width. Stand on the balls of your feet, feet and knees facing out to the sides, heels together. Keep your back erect if you can, and shoulders relaxed and even. Lift your head high, as if you were a prima ballerina.* ▲

Tighten your behind and tip your pelvis up as high as you can. Return your pelvis to the straight starting position. Lower your body an inch, still keeping heels together and balancing on toes. Remember: Do not stick out your behind. That puts pressure on the lower back. ▲

Repeat the above process, tipping your pelvis forward and moving it back, then lowering your body another inch. Do combination again lowering 1 inch more. Shoulders should be as even as you can keep them and, if you have to hold onto the barre tightly, that's all right. Reverse the process until you have returned to your middle position. Do this combination 2 more times. When your legs are strong enough, you will be able to stand up straight. ▲

Note: *Each combination of moving the pelvis up and back and lowering your body counts as 1 movement.*

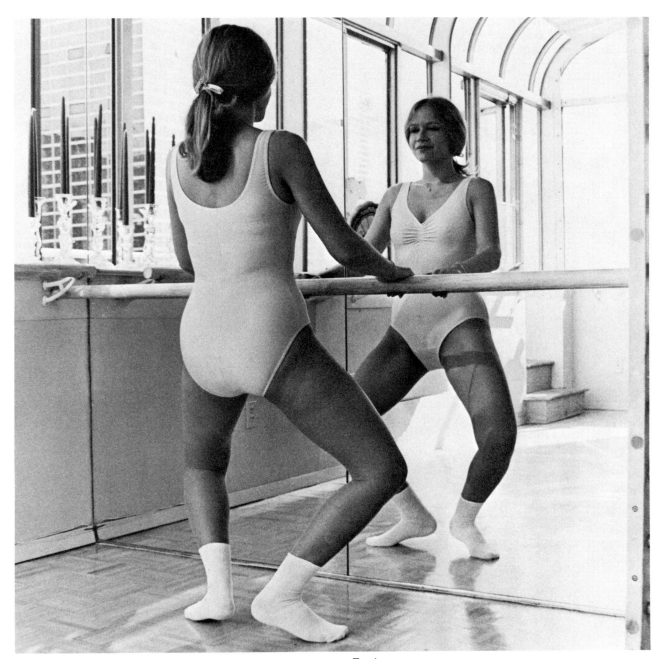

FOR THE LEGS #2 *Facing the barre, hold on with both hands at shoulder width. Go up on the balls of your feet, knees and feet facing outward, heels together. Keep your back straight, if possible. Hold your head high. Lower your body 3 inches and no more. Do not drop your heels. Keep your body straight. Go back to your original position and repeat for a total of 10 times.* ▲

Do not attempt the next two exercises if you have a tendency toward sciatica syndrome.

FOR THE LEGS #3 Note: *Do not force your leg higher than it can easily reach.* See stretch #1 in Chapter 12. *Put your left heel up on the* barre—*or whatever you are using as a* barre—*with your body sideways. Stretch your arms up toward the ceiling, stretching your abdominals. Turn body toward your foot. Remember: Do not put your foot on something too high to keep your balance.* ▲

With arms outstretched, continue to lean your torso over your leg. Keep back stretched toward your raised foot. Beware that you do not lock your knees. ▲

Rest your hands across the shin of your raised leg, as close to your foot as you can comfortably reach. Gently move your torso a quarter of an inch toward your knee and back. Do 50. If you already feel a strong stretch, do not move. Simply hold that stretched position for a count of 50. Keep your entire body relaxed. Repeat with other leg. Do not force knee down with your hands. Don't worry if you can't straighten your raised leg. Bending like this is fine. Your leg will straighten when it is ready. It does not need your assistance. ▲

FOR THE LEGS #4   *Raise your right leg to the* barre, *placing the arch on the* barre. *Hold the* barre *with your hands on both sides of the foot, bending the right knee. Scoot forward with your left foot from 1 to 5 inches.* ▲

Straighten your raised leg as far as possible without pulling on the barre *with your hands. You should only use the* barre *for balance. Do not lock your knees on either leg, and do not force your raised leg to straighten. When your hamstrings are ready, you will be able to do this with ease. Hold for a count of 50. Repeat on the other side.* ▲

CHAPTER TEN

For the Behind and Hips

I had to fight the temptation to call this chapter "Gone with the Goosh" because that is exactly what happens when you do these exercises.

I've never kept a written record of the complaints my new students have about their bodies, but if I did, nine out of ten would be about their hips and behinds. You will be surprised at how conscious of your own behind and hips you become once you begin these exercises. I know of one student who missed a bus because she had become so preoccupied with studying the reflection of her pretty new shape in a nearby window.

I continually warn students not to invest money in expensive clothes for the time being. When their hips start pulling in and their behinds move in and up, their inner thighs also become smaller. In short, their whole proportion changes. Turn back to the Portfolio of Proof (Chapter 4) if you have any doubts. When your body changes shape like this, the cut of your slacks must change as well.

Most of the popular pants designed for American women are cut to cover the wide hips and pear-shaped spread that is so prevalent today. Once you have gotten your slim, tight hips and high, young-looking behind, you will find that your favorite pants' label is now your *former* favorite. You will have a grand time trying on different styles of clothes and noticing your body's wonderful new curves.

Even my male students (some in their early twenties) are excited by the changes in their derrières. They will get fast results from these exercises, but it won't look as dramatic as

This is the perfect bottom line—drawn front to back, level from the pubic bone to the rear. It runs just below the hip joints, highlighting both hips and behind. See how my behind is firm and round? It's even higher than the line. This is what you see people comparing in the mirrors when they think no one is looking. If your behind drops below this imaginary line in back, you know you have to get to work on tightening the muscles and lifting everything, as I have done. ◄

it does for women, yet they feel it just the same.

These exercises work because they concentrate on the very muscles you must tighten to have thin thighs and a well-shaped behind. I see no reason to spend time doing one set of exercises for the behind and another for the hips when this one group of movements will:

● Resculpt the behind.
● Round and lift the buttocks.
● Restore firmness.
● Erase saddlebags.
● Tighten inner thighs.
● Develop the behind without harming the lower back.
● Stretch the spine.

In addition, these exercises allow you to use your arms and upper back just enough to make them beautiful. You will find that none of the movements I teach will add bulk to your arms and shoulders. Instead, they tighten to give you that youthful, firm look. It only seems like magic.

New students actually laugh at their legs in disbelief when they find that they are unable to lift them off the floor. They tell me there's no way they can move them back and forth. I remind them to talk sweetly to their muscles and to keep trying. Keep concentrating. You'll be able to do it sooner or later.

If you have positioned your body correctly, with your hip rolled forward and your pelvis tipped up to the front, you may have some difficulty in coordinating these tiny little movements. Once you have taught your body to accept this as a natural position, your movements will become easy and your muscles will respond automatically for you.

I have seen long lists of exercises that are supposed to decrease the size of the buttocks—jogging, aerobic dancing, swimming, weights—the works. They may do some good if you are sixteen, but once your body has begun to slip, there is no way that running around a track or jerking your body about to disco music can halt the ravages of time. You need drastic measures: *deep* contractions. Just tightening and releasing your behind muscles is not enough. It is merely preparation for exercise and nothing more.

Soon you will see a true sign of fitness—a slight hollow along the sides of your hips as your thighs and behind are made tighter. Look at a picture of a dancer or gymnast. This little dent is at the juncture of the hip and thigh muscles. When both sets are taut and firm there is a lovely definition that sets them off.

These exercises are so special I have used two models, with two very different body types, to demonstrate how to do them. Lane, the little blonde, is my twenty-one-year-old niece. Like me, she has scoliosis and swayback and, as a child, had the same problems with her legs and feet as I did. I had shown her the exercises several years ago. She only did them when her back hurt, but she never did the program seriously until she visited me in New York. She took only two classes and was photographed for the book!

Shelly is in her forties. This mother of a teenage daughter is one of those rare people who was *born* with a nice, tight body. However, one morning in her late thirties, Shelly woke up and saw nothing but goosh . . . almost overnight. Since then, she has exercised with me on and off for a year.

Note: *The mistake everyone makes at first is the failure to tighten behind muscles and curl pelvis up, keep arms straight, hips even, back erect, and stomach in. Do not arch back or stick behind out.* ◄

FOR THE BEHIND AND HIPS
#1 *Facing the barre, sit on the right side of your derrière. Right leg is positioned in front of you, bent at the knee, so that the right heel is even with your crotch, 8 or 10 inches from your body. The left leg is extended to the left, bent backward at the knee. The knee is even with the left hip and the left foot is behind you and relaxed. Hold barre with your right hand and rest left hand on left hip to ease it forward. Roll the left hip forward, pointing your left knee into the floor. Your foot will start to come off the floor.* ◄

Without letting your hip roll back, put your left hand on the barre. Try to tighten your behind and tip your pelvis up. Try to keep your back straight. At first you may lean over and hold on to the barre for dear life, but once your behind muscles learn to work and become stronger, you will merely use the barre for balance, if at all. ▶

Lift left knee not more than 3 inches off the floor, keeping the knee turned to the floor and the foot up. Move raised leg back one-half inch, without letting your hip or pelvis change position. Slowly return your left knee one-half inch to its original position even with left hip. Gently move leg back and forth like this, 100 times on each side. I suggest that you do 20 on one side, switch, and do 20 on the other, back and forth. Work up to 100 on each side. If you feel too tired or are too uncomfortable to continue, take breathers. Do as many as you can. If you have raised your knee too high, you will throw your hip back and transfer the control to your front thigh muscles instead of letting your behind do the work. If you feel an ache going up your hip to your waist, either lean over to the opposite side, or switch sides to release it. There is nothing wrong. Your muscles are simply weak in the beginning. ▶

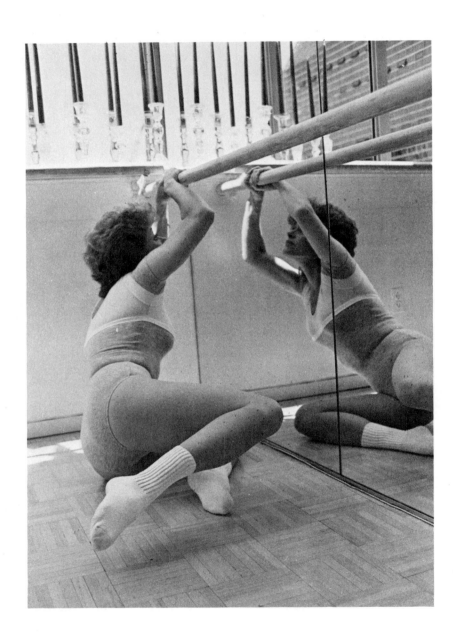

THE ALMOST WRONG WAY
Don't be upset if you start out in this position. Most people do. When your behind muscles get tighter, you will be able to sit up much straighter. People with especially weak behind muscles may need to hold the barre with their hands close together on one side in order to maintain balance. The important thing is to do the exercise. Your style will improve as you get stronger. ◀

For the Behind and Hips

FOR THE BEHIND AND HIPS
#2 *After working on your right side, switch to the left to start the second exercise. In the same starting position, straighten the left leg to the left side, resting on the floor.* ◄

Roll your left hip forward, tightening the behind and curling the pelvis up. Try to turn your leg so that your toes are pointed to the floor. Do not lock the left knee. Relax your shoulders. ►

Keep your hip rolled forward and your behind tight. Your pelvis is curled upward. Raise your left leg not more than 3 inches off the floor and return. Just keep at it. Even if you can't lift it off the floor, keep trying. Eventually, it will lift. Do 20, alternate sides, working up to 100 on each side. Look at how rounded Lane's left cheek is

compared to her right. You can actually see how you can look if you do this exercise in front of a mirror, with a second mirror behind you. If you don't have a mirror, feel your contracted behind with your hand to get some sense of how round, tight, and strong your bottom can be naturally. ▲

91

THE BEGINNER'S ALTERNATIVE *When you begin this exercise, you may find that you have to lean over like this, simply to be able to raise your leg. This is perfectly all right for now, if you remember not to continue that way once your muscles are strong enough . . . or you won't get the results you want.* ◄

DRASTIC MEASURES *Shelly demonstrates another way that beginners attempt this exercise. If this is the only way you can get your leg off the floor, do it until you acquire enough coordination to do it properly. Know, however, that if you do the exercise this way, you use your thigh muscles more than your hips and behind.* ►

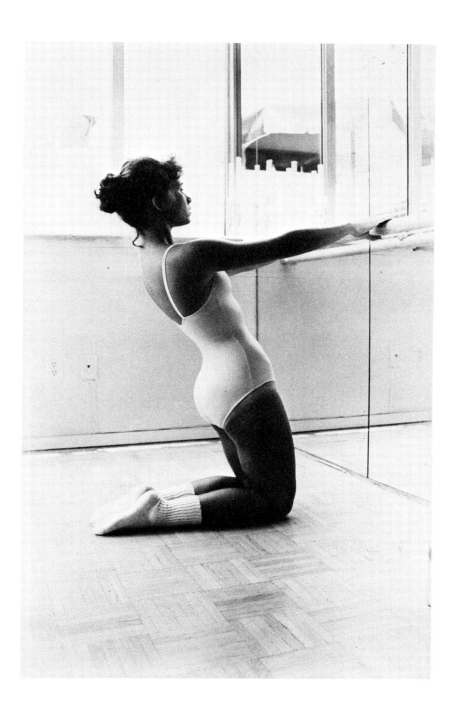

FOR THE BEHIND AND HIPS
#3 *Kneel facing the barre, your knees away from the wall. (Always use padding under your knees for protection.) If you are unable to kneel, see detailed instructions in the Advanced Program, Chapter 22, Exercises #1 and #2. Lean back, so that your arms are straight. Tighten behind and curl pelvis up. This is the foundation for these exercises.* ◄

Round your shoulders forward in order to stretch your spine and keep your elbows straight. You will look and feel as if you are water skiing. It doesn't matter how high or low you hold your arms as long as you are able to lean back with straight arms and your pelvis tipped upward. If you bend your arms, you automatically arch your back and push out your behind. ▲

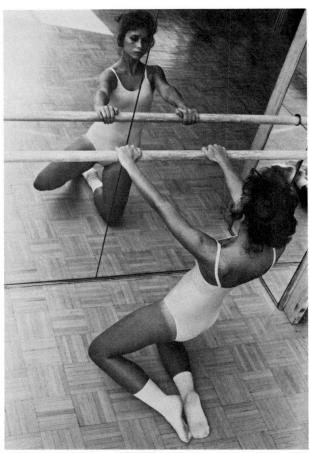

Slowly raise your left knee up to the left side, leaving your foot on the floor beside the right foot. (Because of her scoliosis, Lane has found that the only way she can keep her pelvis tipped is to turn her left hip slightly to one side.) Take the knee up as high as you can until your left foot starts to come off the floor. This is how most of you will do this exercise at first until you learn to keep your hips even. ▲

Raise your left foot 3 inches, 4 at the most, from that position while keeping your pelvis tipped upward and behind tight. Keep your shoulders rounded forward to keep from arching your back. Move knee back a half inch to an inch and return to position even with your right knee. Do 100 on each side, switching when necessary. If you bring your knee too far forward when you return to original position, you release the contraction of your behind muscles, lessening the benefit of the exercise. Until Lane's sacrum area becomes looser, she will not be able to keep both hips even. ▼

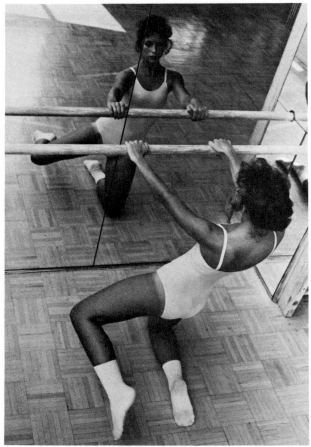

COMMON MISTAKES *Initially, you will be tempted to arch your back, stick out your behind, and bend your elbows. Once you overcome this, it is difficult to do it any other way but properly—your pelvis tipped up and forward, hips even, and shoulders rounded. Shelly had to concentrate to recall what it was like when she started out. She has become so strong and has such control over her movements that she found it difficult to revert to beginner's level for these pictures.* ▶

FOR THE HIPS AND BEHIND
#4   *As in the third exercise, kneel facing the* barre *with your hips even, left leg straight out to the side. Do not lock your knee. Lean back, holding the* barre *so that your arms are straight. Roll your left leg over so that your knee and the top of your foot face the floor, if possible. Relax and concentrate your energy on the part of the body involved.* ▲

Without shifting the position of your hands on the barre, *pull your left leg to the right, toward your body, without bending your leg. Ease over onto the side of your right knee to lessen pressure there. Now tighten your behind and tip your pelvis up, more than you think you can. Round shoulders forward.* ▲

We are in the "Decade of the Derrière." A Syracuse University sociologist reported that American women and men are more concerned with their hips and rear ends than with the bustline. However, with all this attention, many beautiful women have let their buttocks lose their peachlike roundness, settling for a pear-shaped bulge. I know that it is possible for anyone, regardless of age, to have a high, childlike behind and trim hips. ▼

Without allowing your leg to turn upward, move foot and leg up and down, not more than 3 inches. Raise your leg and put it back to the floor 100 times with each leg—50 left, 50 right, 50 left, 50 right. Again, you will find it difficult in this position at first. However, if you talk to your muscles, coax them to cooperate, you will be able to master this move. Lane is not yet strong enough to do this without turning her leg over a bit. Warning: You are not trying to see how high you can raise your leg. Do not bend elbows and lean into the barre or arch your back and stick out your behind. ▲

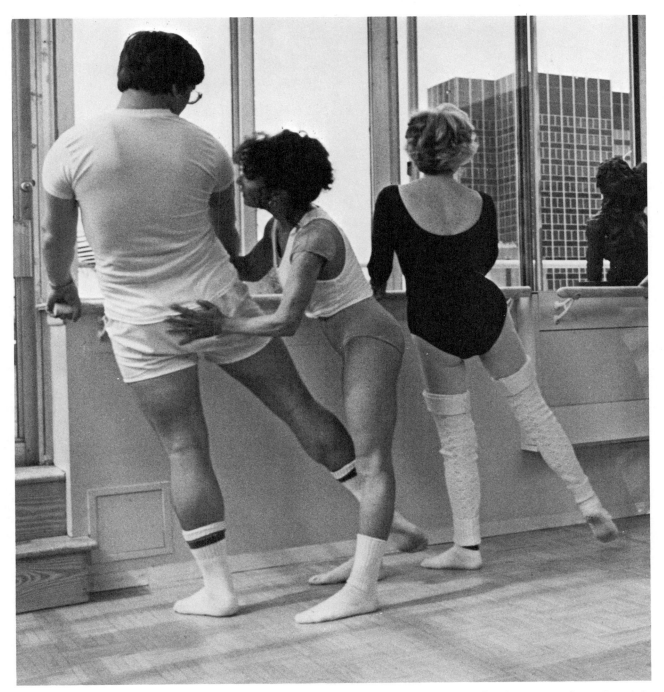

This exercise only appears simple. It is excellent for tightening and shaping the behind and hips and for stretching the lower back. It also contracts your stomach muscles.

Students must learn to rotate their hips forward and tip their pelvises up for proper deep contraction of the muscles that make up the hip and behind. Hips should be kept even, parallel with the barre. ▲

CHAPTER ELEVEN

Open & Close

*T*his is one of the most difficult exercises I teach, and it is also one of my favorites. Whenever I fall into a low-energy slump, I do fifty of these and it makes me feel as if I've had four hours of restful sleep. The results are incredibly fast because you are using several sets of muscles—from your chest, upper back, arms, stomach, abdomen, and even your thighs. At first you will only feel this in your thighs. However, the stronger your thighs become, the more you will notice how much your stomach has been working all along.

By sitting as you do with shoulders against the wall and behind five or six inches from the baseboard, you stretch the muscles up and down your spine. If you feel pressure in your lower back, lean your head forward, putting your chin to your chest, to release the tension in your spine. You may also lean against a sturdy chair or counter and grasp the top with your hands.

Jane, whom you see on these pages, was in a terrible automobile accident that left her unable to work, much less exercise. During the better part of her two-year convalescence, she was in pain and could not exercise. Only two months before these photos were taken, this forty-nine-year-old mother of four college-age children began to exercise again. Because of her medical history, I would not allow her to do this exercise without her doctor's approval. I was completely unaware that she was doing them on her own.

I wasn't surprised, however, when she told me how much better her back had begun to feel.

Anything is possible, as they say! I had been holding Jane back, solely because of my own fears of back pain.

When I show new students after their first class how they will be able to do this Open & Close hanging from the barre after 5 or 6 lessons (if their wrists are strong enough), they are very impressed by the physical strength required to support the body against gravity. ▲

Sit with your shoulders against the wall—or the back of the couch, counter, or bureau front—so that your behind is about 5 or 6 inches from the surface. Reach your arms over your head and hold the edge, if there is one. The height of whatever you are using does not matter. With your legs together, bend them at the knees and pull up to your chest, leaving your toes on the floor. ▶

Clasping the barre firmly with both hands, relax your shoulders and neck. Lift your legs out straight in front of you, as far off the floor as you can hold them. The higher you can hold your legs, the more your stomach muscles will work, which means you'll see and feel results faster. If you feel pressure in your lower back, let your head gently roll forward and rest your chin on your chest. ▶

Open and close your legs, trying not to let them fall to the floor. Concentrate on keeping your neck and shoulders relaxed. Breathe normally. If at first you can't get your legs off the ground, much less make them move, don't worry. Drag them along the floor as you attempt to lift them. Bend your legs if you have to. As you get stronger, you'll be able to straighten them out. Do 4 sets of 5. Increase as you feel stronger. ▶

CHAPTER TWELVE

Stretching

Now you can stretch. Your muscles have been warmed up, even stretched, and put to work. They are ready to be stretched to keep them flexible. Stretching now lengthens muscles after they have been contracted. This is what prevents bulk.

I have positioned this stretching routine toward the end of the One-Hour Program rather than with the Warm-Ups because now is when you need them. You have been pushing your body. It needs the relaxation that stretching brings.

Stretching is essential to an exercise program. It not only helps to keep you flexible, but also to prevent common injuries, such as shin splints or Achilles tendinitis from jogging, or sore shoulders and elbows from tennis. It helps to improve your posture. Stretching is simple. It is not stressful. Done incorrectly, however, it can do more harm than good.

I tell my students to caress their muscles. Be gentle, kind, and respectful to them. I constantly remind them to let their bodies determine how far they stretch. Never *ever* compare your stretches to another person's. If you have to study any living creature, look at animals. Watch a cat or a dog. My students have my cats for inspiration. Pets instinctively know how much to stretch. They are spontaneous, never over-stretching, never jerking or forcing their bodies into position.

Use the time you spend stretching to be alone with your body. Think positive, peaceful thoughts. Relax your spirit *and* your body. Do not *ever* stretch with a partner. Unless you and your partner are professional dancers or athletes,

Keeping my students on their toes mentally as well as physically is important to me. The sculptures all around my studio are the works of my friend Edwina Sandys. Every few weeks I borrow different pieces so there is always something new and exciting to interest the eye. Some are sensuous bodies modeled and cast in bronze. Others are clean-cut from Carrara marble. I do this to remind my students that they are also artists, sculpting their own bodies. ▲

trained to work together, you will not be able to determine the extent of stretch the other person has. If he or she is stronger or more stretched than you, or vice versa, someone could be injured. *Never* allow anyone to push your body into position. Only you can know how far your muscles can go.

There is no standard, ideal range of motion for your joints, nor is there a standard or average pattern of muscular stretch. Every body is different, responding with its own non-standard degree of readiness.

I chose a new student who had completed only one class to demonstrate the stretches I teach *specifically* because she has limited stretching ability. Were I to have an advanced student in the photos, who is as limber as a willow, those of you who are not stretched out, or who are unable to reach or stretch as far as she, would be totally intimidated.

The model, Ellen, is a thirty-two-year-old massage therapist. Her shoulder and arm muscles are very tight from her daily work on patients. Until she started my classes, she had not been able to find an exercise program that would fit into her busy schedule. Once she masters the exercises, she can do them anywhere, anytime.

During stretching, which could easily be called "joint preparations," you pull the connective tissue (fascia) which surrounds your muscles, as well as your muscles and the tendons themselves. If this tissue is not adequately stretched, it shortens. This not only limits movement, it also causes muscles to look knotty and bulky.

Each section of exercises contains stretches that complement the deep contractions you are doing. This special stretching routine completes the program. Move in TRIPLE slow motion.

Stretching is *not* an activity that stands alone. It must be integrated into the total program, largely because, in its function of relaxation, it provides a balance for your body. It gives your body a break. It contributes absolutely nothing toward aerobic fitness or muscle strengthening. If anyone says you can tighten your figure through yoga, or any other regimen that is 90 percent stretching, laugh and leave. There is no way that would work. It is physically impossible. You need the balance of deep contractions and complete stretches to bring your body into shape.

STRETCH #1 *(Stretches inner thighs, hamstrings, lower back, neck, across shoulder blades) (This stretch substitutes for the leg exercises for people with tendency toward sciatica.) Sit on the floor, your legs as far apart as you can take them without upsetting your balance. Place your hands behind your hips, palms down and fingers out. Push your pelvis into the floor and keep your body relaxed. Concentrate on relaxing your legs, putting the energy of the stretch into your pelvis and inner thighs. Don't worry about pointing your toes. Keep your feet and toes relaxed at first.* ◄

Continuing this stretch to the front, rest the palms of your hands on the tops of your thighs to keep the lower back relaxed. Keep your pelvis pushed into the floor. Round your shoulders and push your elbows out to the sides. Lean forward as far as you can and hold that position for 30 seconds, then gently move a quarter of an inch to an inch further, depending upon your flexibility. Move back and forth from that position very slowly and very gently 50 times. If you are doing this for your legs, do 100. If you are very stretched in the back and shoulders, you may be able to start this movement with your hands below your knees or gently on the floor way out in front of you between your legs. Do not grab your ankles or legs or you may pull yourself over too far instead of encouraging your muscles to stretch at their own level. ◄

STRETCH #2 *(Stretches inner thighs, spine, hamstrings, shoulder blades, and back and sides of torso) Starting as you would for the first stretch, remembering to keep your pelvis pushed into the floor, turn your body to one side from the waist. Your chin should be facing your foot. Reach down your leg, placing your hands across the leg as close to your ankle as you can. Round your shoulders and push your elbows out to each side. Your goal: to take your forehead to your knee. Hold for 30 seconds, then move a quarter of an inch to an inch further. Move back and forth from that position 50 times. Return to an upright position and then gently turn to the opposite side and repeat.* ▲

STRETCH #3 *(Stretches the spine, shoulder blades, hamstrings, calves) Sitting upright with your feet and legs together in front of you, relax your legs so that your feet are in a neutral but upright position. Do not lock your knees or push them into the floor. Round your shoulders and place your hands across your legs as low as you can reach. (Do not put your hands across your knees as this could force them downward and may damage the joints.) Your goal is to touch your head to your knees. Stretch over as far as you can. Hold for 30 seconds and, once again, move a quarter of an inch to an inch further. Move back and forth from there 50 times. If you lean your head forward, chin to chest, you will also benefit from a well-stretched neck.* ▲

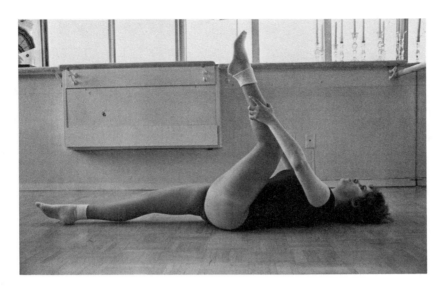

STRETCH #4 *(Stretches the hamstrings, spine, neck, and across shoulder blades) Lie flat on the floor on your back. Straighten your neck and lift your chin toward the ceiling. Concentrate on relaxing your* shoulders. *Bring your left leg up and grab the back of your knee or calf, whichever is more comfortable. Do not force your raised leg to straighten. Bend your elbows out to the sides and hold this position for 30* seconds. *Gently ease your raised leg toward your chest a half inch to an inch closer and move back and forth in a delicate, slow movement. Do 50 and repeat with the other leg.* ▲

STRETCH #5 (Note: *This is a wonderful stretch for the lower back. Stretches spine, upper back, between the shoulder blades, pectorals, behind, hips, outer thighs, and lower back) Lie flat on your back, legs together, arms out at shoulder level with your elbows bent at right angles.* Bend your left leg at the knee and bring it over your right leg, keeping legs relaxed and elbows on the floor. Gently try to bring your left knee to the floor, as close to your right elbow as you can go. Switch sides. Do 50 on one side and 50 on the other. During Ellen's first class, she could not touch the floor with her foot. During this photo session she could, and her knee was much lower to the floor than before. I always do this stretching exercise after I have worn heels, even half-inch heels, to untwist my body and even up my hips. ▲

STRETCH #6 *(Stretches the calves, hamstrings, inner thighs, and spine—when done correctly)* Stand facing a wall or barre, *an arm's length away,* and place your hands on it at waist level, if possible, but no higher than shoulder level. Step back 1 foot. Keep your feet together, facing the wall. Relax your shoulders and arms and keep your elbows straight. ◄

Without moving your left leg, lift your right knee to a height midway between the groin and knee of your left leg. Push your left heel into the floor. Tighten your behind and tip your pelvis upward. Gently move your pelvis and hips forward as a unit, keeping your elbows straight but not locked. Do not stick behind out. The lower part of your right leg and your foot should be relaxed. (Gravity will pull them toward the floor.) Do not jerk or bounce your body or force your body weight into the wall. Do 50, then repeat, standing on your right leg with your left leg raised. The result is a thorough, balanced stretch with no damage to the shoulders, elbows, or wrists. A variation of this stretching exercise is done on steps or a curb. I used to teach it that way, but decided that the foot-on-the-floor method is superior because it not only stretches the calves, but also gets to the inner thighs and complete spine as well.

Stretches, like all the exercises I have included in my program, must be done precisely and gently. I can always tell if someone has taken aerobic dancing—they are maniacs with their bodies. ◄

CHAPTER THIRTEEN

For the Pelvis

*I*f you have ever watched a Middle Eastern dancer perform, you will know right away where this series of exercises comes from. I learned them from a belly dancer!

From these people I discovered that anyone, even someone with back problems such as mine, can have a limber, flexible spine and a loose, sensuous pelvis.

In the fifties, when the Hula-Hoop was the rage, thousands of people suffered from many different kinds of disc problems, all stemming from twisting and turning their bodies like maniacs. However, for *centuries*, Middle Eastern dancers—men and women alike—have circled their hips in endless, sultry sweeps without harm. These two movements are basically the same. How, then, did the swivel-hipped fiends of the fifties hurt themselves so hideously?

It was common sense to me: Those elegant, exotic dancers who move like Salome discarding her seven veils, control and coordinate every click, twist, and swirl of their bodies with deliberate, precise grace. They know what they are doing . . . and why. Every little move has a reason. It is a very *powerful* feeling to have control over this part of your body in this way.

To learn these movements, concentrate on your pelvis. Isolate the muscles in that area. Slowly and deliberately, rotate your pelvis in a full, glorious circle. Don't stick out your stomach and then poke your behind in the opposite direction, or simply move your hips from side to side. Visualize a circle. Picture having complete control over your body as you move in a circle.

As you practice the movement patterns outlined in the following chapter, you will realize that subtle movements like these strengthen the back. But the real payoff comes from the development of the inner thighs and pelvic muscles, which will enhance your sexual enjoyment. ▶

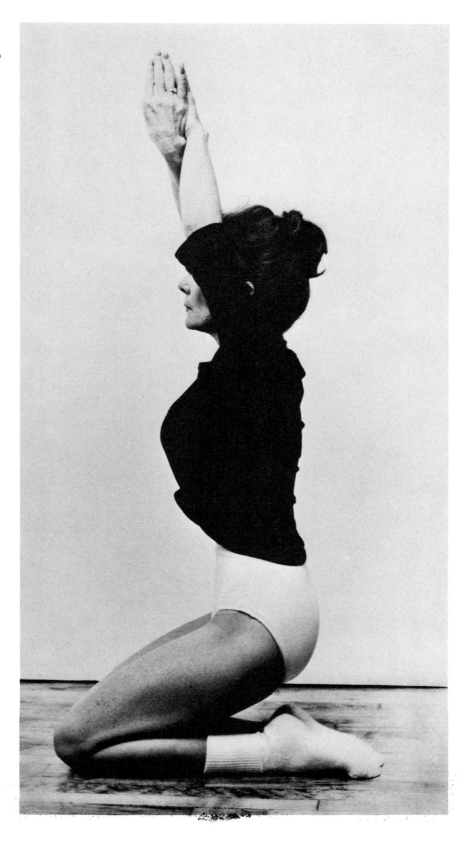

In no time your pelvis will flow with graceful, soft movements. Of all the exercises I teach, these are the ones that both men and women put their hearts and souls into. They learn them quickly and enthusiastically, and tell me that they practice them at home.

This series of exercises works on the behind, thighs, inner thighs, lower back, and the stomach. The Pelvic Rotations stretch your thighs completely, while the Pelvic Scoop contracts them totally. The final stretch works on the thighs and stomach to complete the sequence.

Do these exercises in front of a mirror, even if you must kneel on the bed to see yourself. Try it. Watch how your body moves.

If your calves hurt at first, you need to stretch them more. You may have been wearing high heels and using your calves when you walk. To ease this ache and add stretch to your calves, simply bring your arms in front of your body, rounding your back, as you do the movements.

Hold your head high. Stretch your arms over your head or hold them out to each side. You may even want to put them on your hips. Do whatever makes you feel wonderful.

Once you have perfected the basic movements and are able to perform them with ease, you may want to turn on some sensuous music and move your body in time with it. Now, *you* will be in control of what your pelvis is doing. You'll be surprised at how much strength you have.

Anna, who demonstrates the exercises in this section, is a New York businesswoman in her early forties. When she took her first series of classes with me several years ago, she was under treatment for tachycardia (sudden attacks of rapid heartbeats). She had a nice, but flabby body. Because of her heart condition, I would not let Anna do more than five minutes at her first class. At the second class, she did ten minutes. We increased the time five minutes per class until, as her strength improved, she was able to do the entire routine.

After Anna shaped up, she stopped classes. She resumed classes two years later and had completed two sessions when we took these photos. She was so strong, her body grew noticeably tighter by the hour.

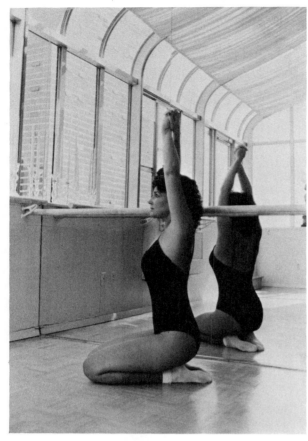

PELVIC ROTATIONS *Sit back on your heels. Stretch your arms over your head. Lift your head and torso high, stretching upward so that you feel you are 2 inches taller than you really are. Feel your abdomen stretch. To protect your knees, kneel on a pillow or cushion that is large enough to pad both feet and knees.* ▲

Raise your body 3 inches off your heels. Stretch straight up. Then take your hip to the right as far as you can, while maintaining your stretched position. Your arms and head should be held high. ▼

Continue to slowly move your pelvis to the front in a circular motion. Pretend you are stirring a pot of soup with your pelvis. Your body will be farther off your heels than when you started with your pelvis tipped to the front. ▼

Still stretching your body upward, move your pelvis to the left side as far as possible. Keep your knees together and hips even. Now, take your behind to the back, your buttocks over your heels, to complete the circle. Complete 5 circles to the right and reverse. (You can also do 10 Figure 8 rotations.) This loosens your pelvic girdle and stretches your thighs. ▲

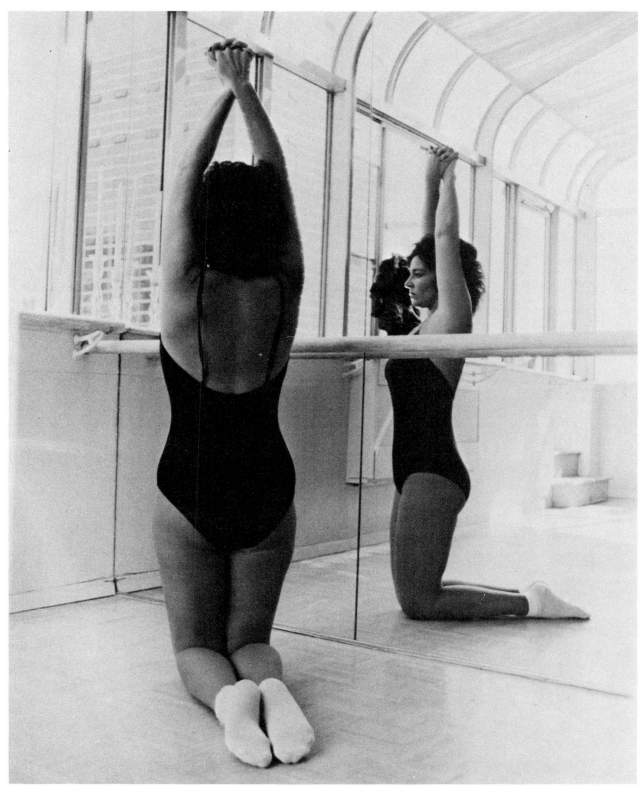

THE PELVIC SCOOP
Kneeling, knees and feet together and arms crossed high *over your head, stretch your torso up as far as you can. If you have pressure on your* *calves, round shoulders and stretch arms forward. (Pretend you are diving into a pool.)* ▲

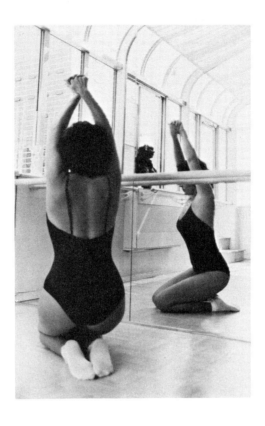

Keep your body straight. Your arms are stretched over your head or, if you prefer, on your hips. Lower your behind in slow motion, aiming it toward your heels. As you feel your behind brush your heels, tighten your behind muscles and slowly tip your pelvis up. Hold for 2 seconds, keeping your pelvis up. ▶

Keeping your knees together and pelvis tipped upward, gently scoop *your pelvis up, lifting your body with the strength of your inner thighs and pelvis, to the original kneeling position. Remember to keep stretching your torso. All movements are slow and graceful. Do 10.* ◀

THE THIGH STRETCH
Kneeling with your knees and feet together, put your palms on the floor either beside or behind your toes. Tighten your behind and stomach. Slowly tip your pelvis up as high as you can go. Hold for a count of 10, trying to go higher at each count, then relax. Do 10 times. This also stretches your neck, pectoral muscles, spine, and stomach, as well as your thighs. This stretch does not tighten the behind. ▲

CHAPTER FOURTEEN

Inner Thigh Squeeze

*I*f your legs look wonderful but your inner thighs jiggle when you walk, you are not alone. Inner thighs and underarms are the most difficult areas of the human body to firm up.

I cringe at the very thought of the time and energy wasted on exercises that are supposed to tighten the inner thighs and don't. Especially since I've found an exercise that works. In fact, it works so well I wouldn't teach anything else.

Pay special attention to this area of the upper leg because, as the *outer* thigh becomes tighter, the *inner* thigh will appear to be flabbier and fleshier than ever before.

My primary objection to other inner thigh exercises is that they are incomplete. Most are stretches without the all-important balancing action of a contraction. Unless your muscles are contracted, you will have well-stretched legs with mushy, dangling inner thighs.

This is a peaceful exercise—a perfect way to end an exercise session. It can be done wherever you can sit on the floor, spread your legs out straight in front of you, and squeeze the sides of a chair, table, or ladder—whatever you have handy. Just make sure it's not your great-grandmother's Queen Anne lady's desk chair or anything else that is fragile. Many chair legs have been broken by inner thighs so strong that the deep contraction crushes the furniture.

When deciding what you should squeeze, look for a chair or table with legs between twelve and thirty-six inches apart. The distance does not really matter, but this span is most comfortable.

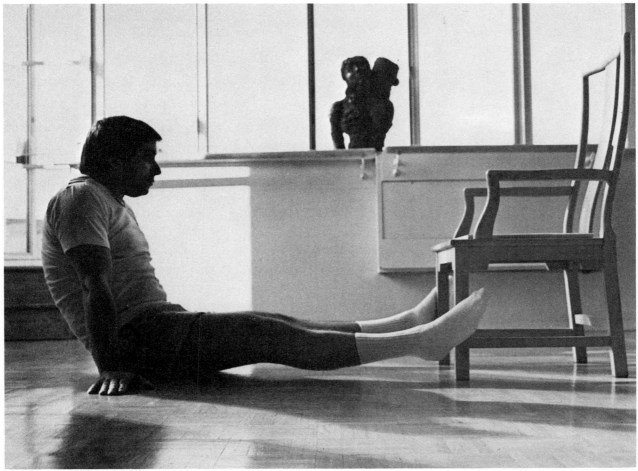

THE MAIN SQUEEZE *Sit on the floor in front of a chair, legs out in front of you. Place the arch of each foot on the outside of the chair legs, pointing your toes as though trying to crush the chair legs together with your feet. Place hands gently on the floor beside your hips or slightly forward. Relax the top of your* *body and let your head and shoulders fall forward so as not to put pressure on your lower back. Squeeze your feet and legs together around the chair legs, tightening your inner thighs as much as you can for a slow count of 100. Hold steadily; do not squeeze and release. When you first start this* *exercise, you may feel the muscles in the calves and inner knee areas working. This is because your inner thighs are lazy. They've never worked this hard before, and will let anything do their work for them. Very soon you will only feel it in your inner thighs.* ▲

Harvey, who had been to two classes when these pictures were taken, demonstrates two ways to do this very valuable exercise.

As you can see, we women are not alone in wanting our legs to be firm and fit all over—including our inner thighs.

A VARIATION ON THE MAIN SQUEEZE *The difference here is in the placement of the hands and arms to release your lower back more. Rest your hands gently on the floor between your legs, rounding your shoulders forward so that your hands are even with your knees.*

Whenever you do this powerful exercise, relax your neck, arms, lower back, shoulders— everything but your inner thighs—and think peaceful, positive thoughts. This will make you even more aware that you do not have to put pressure on your lower back. At about *the count of 50, you will feel the shift and your inner thigh muscles will take over. By your third session, you will be counting to 300 before stopping this relaxing squeeze. To accomplish this, count to 100, release, and repeat by 100s. ▲*

CHAPTER FIFTEEN

The One-Hour Program— A Summary

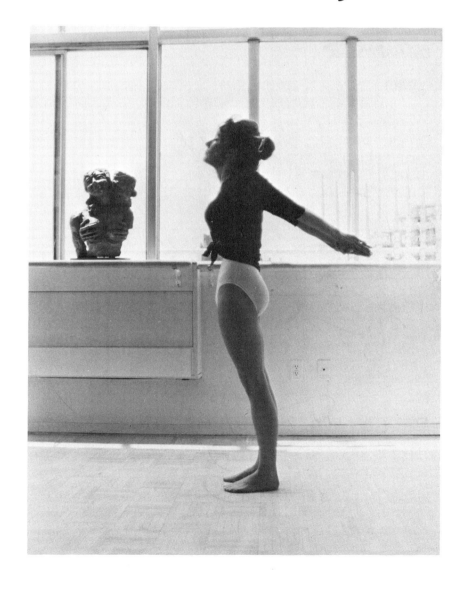

INSTRUCTIONS

This chart can provide you with the cues you need to
guide you through the One-Hour Program. Use the
column at the right to pencil in the number of
repetitions you need to do, or make little sketches
that will tickle your memory about the position you
should be in.

Exercise	Progress / Notes
WARMING UP Warm-up # 1 (Hanging) Warm-up # 2 (Up and Down) Underarm Tightener Waist Stretch Hamstring Stretch Neck Exercise #1 (Roll) Neck Exercise #2 (Side to Side)	
FOR THE STOMACH For the Stomach #1 (Knees Bent) For the Stomach #2 (One Leg Up) For the Stomach #3 (Both Legs Up)	
FOR THE LEGS For the Legs #1 (Up-Back-Down) For the Legs #2 (Up and Down) For the Legs #3 (Heel on *Barre*) For the Legs #4 (Arch on *Barre*)	

Exercise	Progress / Notes
FOR THE BEHIND AND HIPS For the Behind and Hips #1 (Seated, Leg Bent) For the Behind and Hips #2 (Seated, Leg Straight) For the Behind and Hips #3 (Kneeling, Leg Bent) For the Behind and Hips #4 (Kneeling, Leg Straight)	
OPEN & CLOSE	
STRETCHING Stretch #1 (Legs Apart) Stretch #2 (To the Sides) Stretch #3 (Legs Together) Stretch #4 (Hamstring Stretch) Stretch #5 (Leg Over) Stretch #6 (Calves)	
FOR THE PELVIS Pelvic Rotations Pelvic Scoop Thigh Stretch	
INNER THIGH SQUEEZE The Main Squeeze Variation on Main Squeeze	

CHAPTER SIXTEEN

The 15-Minute Maintenance Plan

When I hear someone say they exercise an hour every day to try to get a beautiful figure, I find it difficult not to laugh. If a beautiful body is what they want, these people have the wrong idea about exercise. I don't spend an hour a day on my own body, and exercise is my profession!

Most people don't have the time to exercise for an hour each and every day, or even three times a week, as many people recommend. It is not realistic, especially for busy people who have families to take care of and normal, nine-to-five jobs.

The truth is this: An hour a day does not necessarily keep the flab away.

To promise yourself that you will make this unrealistic demand on your time and your body is setting yourself up for failure. This is especially true if you are doing exercises that do not produce rapid results. Nine times out of ten you will quit exercising altogether if you are unable to maintain this one hour per day regimen for yourself without seeing dramatic and rapid improvements in your body. I've seen it happen too often.

This 15-Minute Maintenance Plan is my answer to the time problems facing today's busy person. I first designed it for my students who travel and don't have time for one-hour workouts. Once students have completed a program of classes and have their bodies looking the way they want them to, they often adopt this as a daily routine.

Do not expect to discontinue the One-Hour Program in favor of this 15-Minute Maintenance Plan until you com-

Before she tightened up her body so much that she no longer wore large-size clothes, Kelle Kerr was a busy model for the larger woman. This snapshot will give you an idea of how hefty she was at her prime as a model. ▲

pletely understand the movements and want to maintain your fitness level. This is *not* a program for beginners. I cannot stress this warning enough.

The 15-Minute Maintenance Plan is an abbreviated version of the One-Hour Program. It is the basics, timed to take fifteen minutes from start to finish.

Should you want to concentrate on a specific part of the body that is not emphasized in this short session, feel free. Add whatever exercises from the One-Hour Program that you feel you should, but also add to your schedule the amount of time that you will need to do them. *Do not* eliminate any exercise simply to allow yourself time to do another exercise within the fifteen-minute time period.

This program is balanced to work on the parts of the body that generally need the most work. To omit one exercise in favor of something else, or something you find easier or more comfortable to do, would upset this balance. You won't get the rapid results you desire.

Break down the 15-Minute Maintenance Plan even further, interspersing your exercises with your daily schedule. One young mother I know works a full-time job. She does five minutes of the exercises in the morning, before she wakes the children for nursery school, and then works in five minutes more at her office, instead of having coffee and danish on her morning break. She completes her program before bedtime, after her little ones have gone to sleep.

One might think she could get enough exercise with her busy schedule, but she can't. By dividing the fifteen-minute program to fit her time requirements, she now has the time to take care of her body *and* do everything else on her daily agenda.

This student decided to take my advice after she had spent hundreds of dollars joining health clubs and gyms. She reasoned that, since she had paid so much to join, she would *make* time to go and work out, but for no other reason than to get her money's worth. She never had the time, no matter how much she juggled her schedule. Now, she gets in an hour and fifteen minutes of concentrated exercise per five-day work week and feels fabulous for it. She knows that she could have faster results in shaping her body if she interspersed the One-Hour Program with the 15-Minute Maintenance Plan every second or third day, but that is not always possible.

Kelle Kerr, who demonstrated these exercises for our photographs, is a model in real life. She was one of the top large-size models in the business when she started coming

129

to my classes to tone up her body. After a very short time, however, she had tightened up so much that she was too small for the job, even though she had not lost any weight.

For a while Kelle was able to continue working with the help of a padded body suit that made her body her pre-exercise size. Before long that didn't work—her neck had become too long and thin, and her legs, too slim and sleek to be in proportion with her padded, larger body.

With her new, voluptuous body, Kelle is getting many new modeling jobs, often more exciting than before.

No matter what other shape-up program Kelle has tried, she invariably comes back to these exercises to keep her body in top form . . . and she doesn't have to take time off from her career to exercise, either.

When you see the exercises in this 15-Minute Maintenance Plan, you may want to refresh your memory with the more detailed instructions in the One-Hour Program.

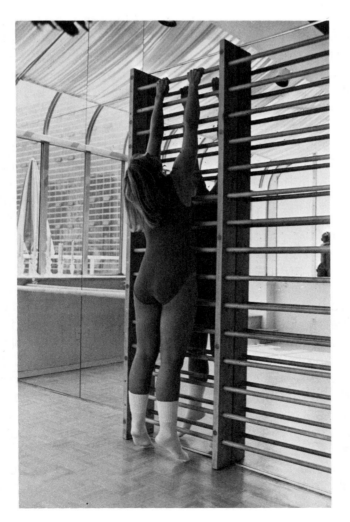

WARMING UP # 1 *Hang from a ladder or door, completely relaxing your body and allowing any tension or stress you may feel to drip like wax to the floor. This stretches the spine and relaxes the body, readying you to begin exercise. Hold for as long as your wrists and arms will allow. The longer you can hang, the stronger your arms and wrists will become and the more your entire body will stretch.* ◄

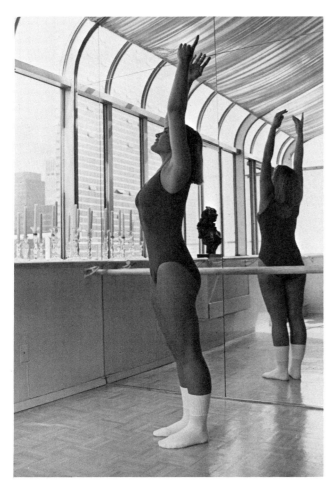

Flex the knees and bend forward, gently moving your arms out in front of you. Be sure to keep stretching out with your torso as you move. Continue to bend your legs and stretch your torso. Hold in your stomach and breathe naturally. Stretch your arms up behind you as far as possible. Do not swing or jerk your arms. Every move must be gentle and precise. Gently move your arms forward again and stretch upward into an erect position. Reach for the sky. Repeat 5 times. ▼

Stand erect, with legs and feet together or no more than a foot apart for balance. Stretch arms up over the head, lifting the torso as high as you can, as if you were trying to make yourself 2 inches taller. ▲

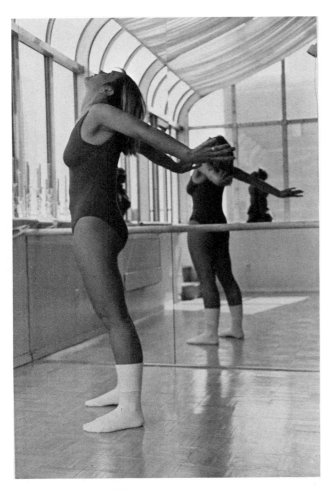

WAIST STRETCH *Stand up straight, placing your left hand on the side of your left leg, elbow out. Tighten your behind muscles and tip your pelvis upward. Keep your tummy tight and your hips even. Stretch your body upward. Reach over your head and to the left with your right arm, keeping your elbow straight and stretching out with your fingers as though you were trying to touch something on a table beside you on the left. Reach as far as you can and then reach a half inch farther. Your left arm will bend as it rests on your leg. Relax neck. Do not bounce and do not throw your hip out if at all possible. Remember: Bring your upper body and arms around to the front before you straighten up. Do 75 on each side.* ▼

FOR TIGHT UNDERARMS
Stand erect with your arms stretched out straight to the sides at shoulder level. Roll arms forward from the shoulder so that your thumbs face upward. Reach your arms to the back, as though trying to lock thumbs. Hold your head and shoulders back to loosen tightness between your shoulder blades and in your pectorals. Gently move arms back and forth a half inch in each direction. Do 75. Remember: Keep your buttocks tight, pelvis tipped up, and hold in your stomach as you do any of these standing exercises. ▲

FOR THE STOMACH #1 *Lie on your back with your knees bent and feet flat on the floor. Push the small of your back into the floor. Grab your inner thighs, elbows out, and gently pull your upper body up as far as you can. Keep your shoulders rounded and relaxed. Raise your arms parallel with your thighs without letting your head and shoulders drop back to the floor. Reach forward from this point a half inch to an inch further. Do not do this exercise by moving your head. Reach with your arms, shoulders, and upper body—rounding upward from just under your bust—as one gentle movement. The behind and legs do not move. Keep them relaxed. Repeat 75 times.* ▲

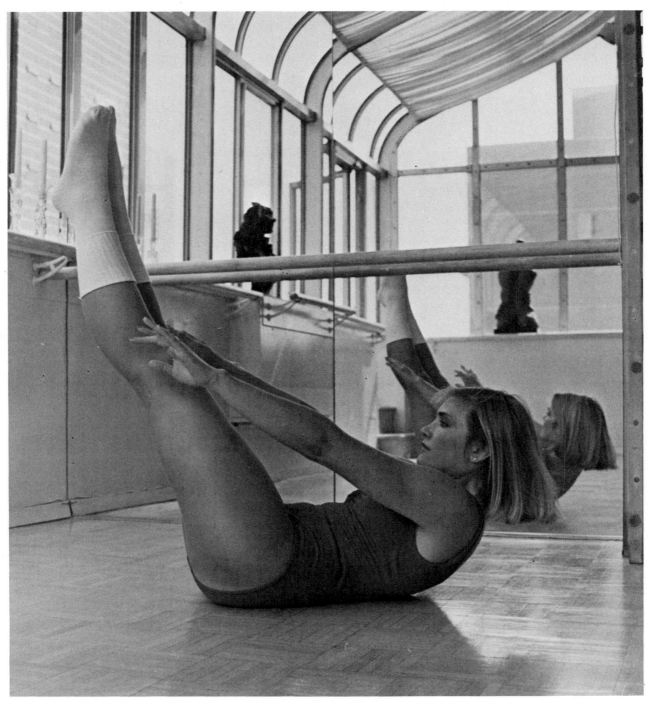

FOR THE STOMACH #2 *Lie flat on your back, pressing the small of your back into the floor, and raise your legs straight upward to at least a 60-degree angle with the floor. Grasp your outer legs as close to your knees as you can reach.*

Extending your elbows out to each side, round your shoulders, and pull the top of your body upward toward your legs. Without dropping your legs and arms or your upper body, release hold on your legs. Reach arms upward, as if

you were trying to touch your toes. Move the top of your body up and down a half inch to an inch in each direction. Repeat 75 times. Return to starting position. ▲

FOR THE LEGS #1 *Stand on your toes, facing the barre, with your heels together, knees and toes turned out to the sides, back erect and stomach in. Relax your shoulders and arms as you gently grasp the barre with both hands. Lift your head high. Imagine you are being seated in a chair. Do not stick out your behind—tighten your buttocks and tilt your pelvis upward. Let your pelvis go back to the starting position. Lower your body not more than an inch, keeping your legs as relaxed as possible and your knees bent, heels touching.* ▼

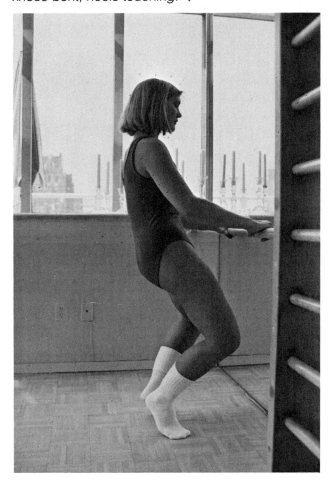

Tilt your pelvis up again and then return to the straightened position, 1 inch lower than when you started this exercise. Lower your body another inch. Repeat this combination 1 more time, lowering your body another inch, and then return to a standing position by reversing the process—tip pelvis upward, back, and then raise your body 1 inch higher, continuing the process until you are at the original starting position. Do 5. Do not let heels go down when reversing the process. ▲

FOR THE LEGS #2 *Stand erect with 1 foot resting gently on the barre. Raise your arms high over your head, stretching your entire body upward. When you put 1 foot up on the barre, you must not lock the knee of the leg you are standing on. Turn your torso forward, bending your body over your raised leg, and stretch your arms gently toward your ankle. Fold your hands across your raised leg, as close to the ankle as possible. Gently lean forward over your leg, holding that position or moving the upper body back and forth, a half inch in each direction, 25 times. Do not jerk. Make slow, precise motions. Change legs and repeat. Remember: People with a tendency toward the sciatica syndrome should ask their physician or chiropractor if they should do this exercise.* ▲

FOR TIGHTENING THE BEHIND AND HIPS #1 *Sit on the floor, facing the barre—or whatever you're using as a barre—with the right leg bent in front of the body and the left leg extended to the side, knee bent so that foot is behind body.*

Clasp the barre with both hands. Roll left hip forward, allowing the left foot to come off the floor. The foot should be turned upward, higher than the left knee. Tighten behind, and tip pelvis up. Lift knee 2 inches

off the floor. Move left leg gently back 1 inch, keeping left hip rolled forward so that both hips are even. Return leg forward 1 inch. Repeat 75 times on each side. Reminder: Do not bring knee in front of hips. ▲

FOR TIGHTENING BEHIND AND HIPS #2 *Sit on the floor, facing the* barre, *in the same position—the left leg stretched out straight to the left side. If you completed the preceding exercise with your left leg working, start this exercise with your left leg bent in front and* your right leg out to give the muscles on your left side a breather. Clasp the barre with both hands. Roll the left hip toward the barre *and tip pelvis up. Try to turn the top of the left foot toward the floor. Raise left leg 1½ to 2 inches off the floor, keeping the leg straight and the* left hip rolled forward. Remember: If you can raise your leg more than 2 inches off the floor, you are throwing your hip out and not keeping it even. This transfers contractions to your front thigh muscles. Repeat 75 times on each side. ▲

STRETCHING #1 *Sit firmly on the floor, legs spread out to each side. Reach both arms out in front of your body and gently stretch as far forward as you can from that position. Rest hands on floor. Move torso back and forth a half inch in each direction 25 times. Do not jerk or bounce. Remember to curve your shoulders forward to stretch your spine more. Don't worry if you still can't touch the floor with both hands. Keep them on your thighs. Some people stretch easier than others.* ▲

STRETCHING #2   *Stretch your legs out in front of you, knees and feet together. Curl your shoulders forward and stretch your entire torso forward gently, as if you were trying to* touch your knees with your forehead. Resting your wrists across your shins for balance, stretch your body as far as you can for a slow, gentle count of 25. Remember: *The straighter you have your legs, the more intense the stretch. This is not a stretch to be lackadaisical about. Warning: No jerking and no fast movements.* ▲

THE PELVIC SCOOP *Kneel on a pad, knees and feet together. Stretch your body upward, lifting your arms high over your head. Do not arch your back. Relax as you do this exercise. From this position,* *slowly aim your behind down toward your heels. Make sure to keep your torso upright, reaching your arms over your head. When you feel your behind brush your heels, tighten your behind muscles* *and slowly tip your pelvis upward, as you "scoop" your pelvis up from this low position to your upright starting point. Move delicately, carefully, and do not jerk your body upward. Do 8. ▲*

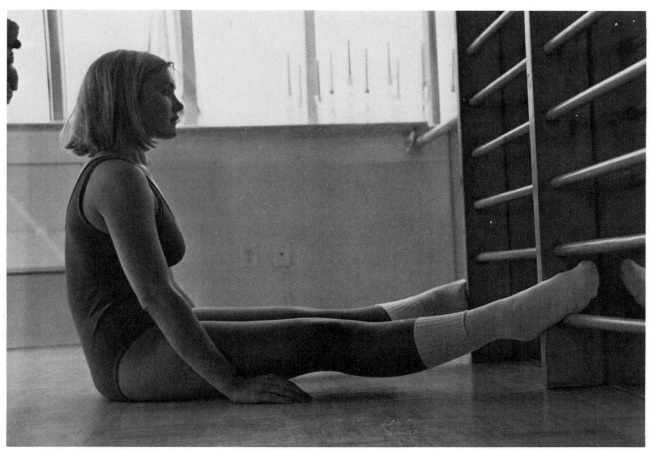

THE INNER THIGH SQUEEZE *Sit on the floor in front of a chair, legs out in front of you. Place the arch of each foot on the outside of the chair legs, pointing your toes as though trying to crush the chair* *legs together with your feet. Place hands gently on the floor beside your hips or slightly forward. Relax the top of your body and let your head and shoulders fall forward a bit to ease back pressure. Squeeze* *your feet and legs together around the chair legs, tightening your inner thighs as much as you can for a slow count of 100. ▲*

CHAPTER SEVENTEEN

It's No Wonder My Back Hurt

*B*eing a nomad for the better part of ten years, everything I owned was either stuffed into, or strapped onto, a rucksack that I carried on my back. For a while I even carried a three-by-five-foot Persian rug with me; at another point, a large African tribal drum.

Often walking great distances between towns, thumbing rides when and where I could, it was sometimes a three-day wait before any means of transportation came my way.

During this time, my sixty-five-pound rucksack and I traveled by bus, train, camel, mule-drawn wagon, and, best of all, by truck. Trucks were preferred, because one could stretch out and sleep in comparative privacy. If I sensed danger, it was not too difficult to roll my pack off and jump out after it.

Most of the time while roaming the world, I weighed less than eighty pounds—especially after several bouts of dysentery. My fragile condition was exacerbated by the constant pain and pressure on my knees, rubbed raw from supporting a weight almost equal to my own for many miles a day. So, between the knees, scoliosis, disc problems, swayback, and distorted feet, it's no wonder my back hurt.

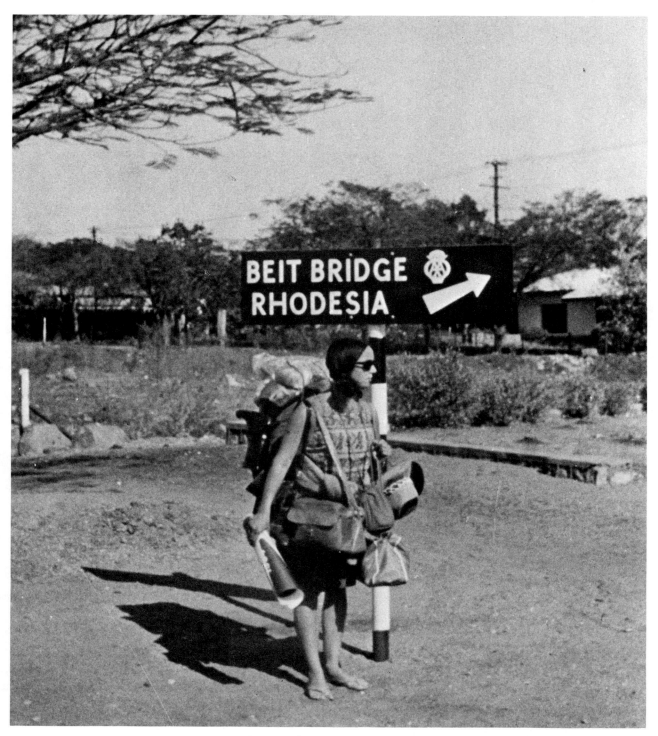

Laden with all my wordly goods, trudging toward Beit Bridge in Rhodesia (now Zimbabwe). I made sure I was clean and tidy so my parents could remember me that way in case I was maimed, raped, or killed—if not all three at once. ▲

CHAPTER EIGHTEEN

Take Care of Your Back

*I*f you have trouble with your back, either from birth defect, stress, illness, or injury, exercise can be your best friend or your worst enemy.

If you do the right exercises, you can improve mobility and minimize pain; if not, you can be in trouble.

Simple stretching exercises, for example, can relax tension in the muscles along the spine. Other exercises can strengthen the abdominal and behind muscles, among others, to provide your spine with additional support.

"Back trouble" is a rather broad term for many very specific problems—a tear or pull of muscle or ligament, a muscle in spasm, compression or degeneration of a disc, degeneration of bone, a curvature of the spine, and even tension. You may even have an infection in some other part of the body that produces what is called a referred pain along the back.

Many of these troubles can be eased considerably, if not reversed, simply by adjusting the way we move. Chronic lower back pain, for example, usually can be alleviated by (1) losing weight, (2) exercising to strengthen the muscles of the pelvic girdle to provide support for this region of the spine, (3) improving posture, and (4) controlling stress instead of letting stress control you.

Who gets back pain is a puzzle. Many people constantly complain of aches and pains, while others live to a ripe old age with scarcely a twinge. It is a bizarre lottery that gives pain to some and none to others.

The way we live almost guarantees that we will have difficulty recovering if we do injure our backs. Our sitting habits, shoes, furniture, the hard pavement of city sidewalks, sports, even emotional stress, come into play, making it practically impossible for us to give our backs time to heal. Everyday tension can put some people into muscle spasms. That's a painful price for the fast pace we live today.

Even in the midst of our ever-growing fitness craze, we lay ourselves open to back injury by some of the very exercises we do to strengthen and stretch our bodies. A certain amount of exercise—besides walking to the kitchen or car—is essential to maintaining muscle tone and cardiovascular fitness, not to mention burning off calories.

The most prevalent problem lies in selecting the most beneficial exercises suitable for people with back problems, or potential back problems. Each of the exercises in this chapter, as well as in the One-Hour Program, come from my own experience. Tobi, the student demonstrating these exercises, is a thirty-four-year-old mother with a seven-year-old son. She has scoliosis—which you can detect in the stretch she does from the chair—and a slight swayback. She is so strong, however, from these exercises, that she is now almost completely into the regular program, with few of the modifications you will see in this chapter. It took her only three classes of special exercise before she was able to move into the regular routine.

Scoliosis is a lateral curvature of the spine creating asymmetry and an "S" or a "C" curve that is visible from behind. Lordosis (swayback) is, simply explained, a "C" curve of the spine when viewed from the side, which forces the stomach forward, no matter how thin a person is.

Parents can check for the signs of scoliosis in their children at an early age—the best time to treat the condition. Have your child bend as if ready to dive into a swimming pool. The back should be bare, so that the spine is visible. Look for a lack of symmetry, such as a twist to one side or the other, a protruding muscle or shoulder blade, or one hip, shoulder, or shoulder blade higher than the other. Females appear at higher risk, but males are far from exempt from the problem.

Detected early, spinal defects such as these can be treated with exercise. This may avert the damage the disorder once caused and avoids crippling in the later years.

Doctors admit that they do not know exactly what causes this problem, but they are finding that the earlier it is detected, the more problems can be averted. Much of the time, exercises that strengthen the muscles along the sides of the spine will be enough to halt the formation of the curvature.

If you detect any problems in your children, see your pediatrician. Ask for a recommendation to an orthopedist who specializes in pediatric bone problems. The progress made in the field is so vast that, detected early, long-range problems can be eliminated. Even people who require surgery, something that is becoming increasingly less frequent, are able to lead active lives whereas in the past they were limited in mobility and flexibility.

The most important part of caring for the back is self-awareness. Pay attention to the signals your body gives you with regard to movement and use. If you detect a pattern of activity followed by pain, consult a physician.

If your physician talks about surgery, ask for and get a second opinion—preferably from someone who is neither a surgeon nor an associate of the first doctor. What you may need is not an operation but, instead, special braces or even a set of stretching and strengthening exercises to free you from the specter of back pain.

When my students see my stomach pushed out, they know I am reverting to my old posture and am not standing correctly. It is impossible for me to stand with my spine straight against the wall. If I press the small of my back to the wall, I must curl my shoulders forward and move my feet out almost a foot. The normal position of the human spine is a relatively straight column with four slight curves: the cervical, at the neck; the thoracic, through the chest; the lumbar, the five vertebrae in the region of the

loins; and the sacrum, the bottom of the spine, where the five sacral vertebrae have become united into a single bone. For me to appear to have a normal posture, I must stand erect, shoulders back, and tighten my behind while tipping my pelvis up. This way, no one will ever know. ◄

Note: All body movements should be done in triple slow motion. Jerking and fast movements can irritate back problems. Key word: gentleness.

EXERCISES I HAVE FOUND TO
BE SAFE FOR PEOPLE WITH
BAD BACKS

To stretch the spine, sit in a chair and lean over with rounded shoulders. This loosens the muscles around the spine just enough to begin other warming-up exercises. ◄

For this spinal stretch, Tobi leans toward a low barre with her feet far enough from the wall to force her to lean forward to hold on. Hold arms straight and relax both arms and legs. Lean back so that the back is completely straight and parallel with the floor. Feet can be apart or together, whichever is more comfortable. Stretch your body away from the barre and hold for a slow count of 25. ▲

This is a version of the waist stretch found in the One-Hour Program. It pulls the side muscles in the lower spine and feels very good. Do this extremely gently and move slowly to the side without jerking up and down. Don't take the body directly to the side. Instead, bend slightly forward. Tighten the behind and tip the pelvis up. Keep the knees relaxed and slightly bent. Rest your right arm, elbow bent, on the upper right thigh. Do 50, building up to 100, on each side. ▼

The difference in the way most people do the underarm exercise and the way I ask Tobi to do it is simple. Knees are bent and feet about a foot apart. The pelvis is tipped up and the behind is tight, helping stretch the spine as well. Lean the head forward, neck relaxed, unless this is uncomfortable; otherwise, hold head straight. Move arms behind body as far as possible, palms up and thumbs as high as possible. Move arms slowly back and forth a half inch. Start with 50 and build to 100. ▲

Begin the hamstring stretch from the One-Hour Program with knees bent, feet about a foot apart. Stretch your arms forward and round your back a little. Tighten your behind and tip your pelvis forward. Relax your legs and neck. Still stretching the spine, bring arms down, dangling them toward the floor. Move the torso up and down a quarter of an inch in each direction or, if that is uncomfortable, just hold. Do 20 without standing up. ▼

Keeping the hips even, turn the upper torso to one side. Bend over and place hands on the upper outer thighs. Then move torso up and down, again moving only a quarter of an inch in each direction. Hold this position if you prefer, or do 20 on each side. When switching sides, do not stretch torso upward again; simply move slowly and gently to the other side. ▲

Lie flat on your back and stretch your arms over your head and your legs straight out as though trying to make your body feel 2 inches longer. In this picture, you can see how Tobi's spine is curved. ◄

Lie on your back, bending your legs at the knees, shoulders flat on the floor. Raise feet off the floor. Lift up your shoulders and head with your hands clasped behind your head, elbows out. Do not tense any part of your upper body as you move your chin toward your chest. Gently lift head and shoulders up a quarter inch and down a quarter inch. Move only from under the bust as you move up and back. Do not jerk. Do not move your head. Also, do not move your behind back and forth. All movements must be in triple slow motion. Do 20 to 50. If your legs feel too heavy and you have no control over them, put your feet up on a chair and lift shoulders up and back in quarter-inch movements. ◄

This variation of the preceding exercise for the stomach calls for you to bend your left leg and place your foot flat on the floor. Stretch your right leg up. Clasp your hands behind your head. Round your shoulders and hold your elbows out to the sides. Raise your head and shoulders off the floor. Move your upper torso up and down a quarter of an inch in each direction, making sure that every movement is gentle and easy. You may bend your raised leg if you wish. Do 20 to 50 on each side. ▲

I consider this to be one of the best back stretches in the world. Lie face up on the floor. Bend arms out at shoulder level, elbows flat on the floor. Bending your right knee, bring it up and over your left leg, as though trying to put your right knee to the floor. If that is impossible, just hold the position, then move your right knee a quarter of an inch farther. Your knee will go lower when it's ready. Do not let your elbows and shoulders come off the floor, if at all possible. Slowly change sides. Do 25 each side. ▲

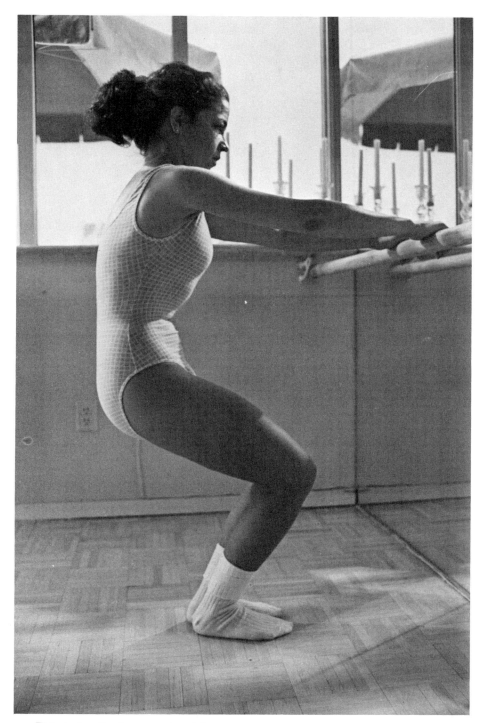

This is for the legs and pelvis and, as a bonus, strengthens the feet and ankles. Stand straight at the barre, clasping it with your hands at shoulder width. Feet are together or as much as 6 inches apart. Tighten behind and tip pelvis upward. Round shoulders and keep your elbows straight. Move pelvis back and forth slowly and gently 10 times. Do not stick behind out. Once you are strong enough, you will be able to go to the exercises in the One-Hour Program. ▲

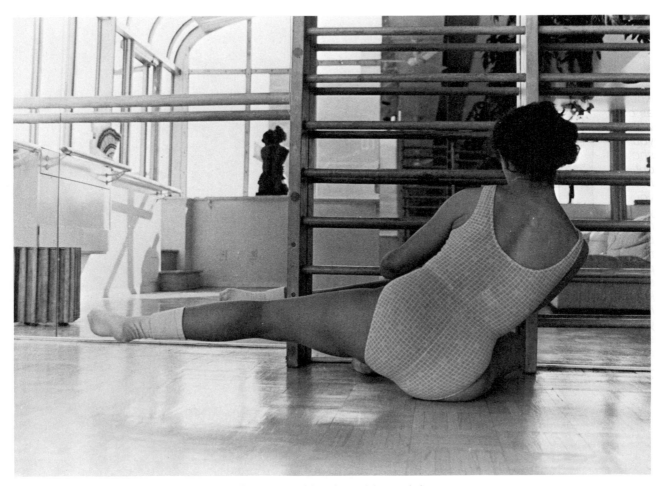

Because of back problems, it is advisable to sit in front of a sturdy chair or low table, with your right leg bent in front of you. Clasp the barre with both hands at waist or chest level. Stretch your left leg out straight to the side. Keep hips even. Raise and lower your leg very slowly not more than 2 inches off the floor. Do 20 on each side, taking your time, building up to 100. It's all right to lean your shoulders to the right to maintain your balance. Concentrate on keeping your behind tight and your pelvis tipped forward and up. As you build strength, you should be able to do the behind and hip exercises from the One-Hour Program. ▲

Kneel on a pad, knees and feet as close together as possible, with your hands on the sides of your waist. Relax your shoulders and hold your elbows out to each side. Slowly aim the behind to your heels, stretching your back without sticking out your behind or arching your back. When you feel your behind touch your heels, gently tighten your behind, tip your pelvis upward very slowly, and scoop upward, returning to the kneeling position. Do 5. If you have any aching in your calves, you can lean forward with your arms, head, and shoulders extended in front, as if you were diving into water. See the Pelvic Scoop in Chapter 13. ▼

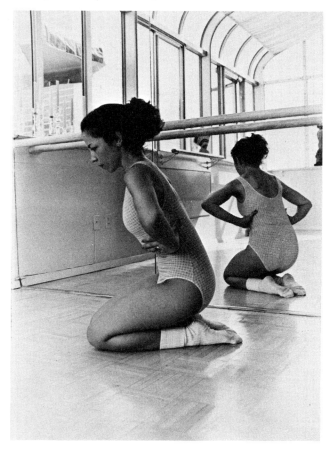

Attempt this only if you have access to a high barre. For people with bad backs, hanging comes as the completion to the exercise program. The muscles are warm and stretched, therefore there is no risk of your becoming too tense—a tendency people have when hanging. As a result of your prior exercises, your back will stretch more fully at the end of the program. If you do this, relax the lower back and pretend your body is like melting wax dripping onto the floor. ▲

CHAPTER NINETEEN

You're Never Too Old to Have a Fabulous Figure

Youth and fitness do not necessarily go hand in hand. However, fitness is definitely a key to having a youthful body, regardless of your age.

Look at Margaret, the student demonstrating the exercises in this chapter. Who would believe she is in her mid-seventies? What is even harder to believe is that she exercises every day—despite the fact that four vertebrae in her neck were surgically fused ten years ago, using bone and tissue taken from her hip, and she has arthritis in her shoulders and back.

"I'm afraid *not* to exercise," she explains. "If I miss one day, I feel intense muscle pain down my spine and I start to stoop over. It sets me back a week."

Despite teasing from her husband and friends, Margaret wears her leotard around the house while doing her housework. "Every time someone calls me I'm on the floor exercising. They think I'm silly, doing this at my age, but I feel great."

She must be in great condition, too. A week before these pictures were taken, she slipped and slid down four carpeted steps, hit a newel-post and fell three feet to the hardwood floor. Her only injury was a massive bruise on her hip and leg, where she landed. You can see it in some of the photos. That is why she is wearing leg warmers.

Falling is one of Margaret's greatest fears, since further injury might break the cervical fusion. Had she settled for a sedentary, overly careful life, doing little physical activity, she would have become a crippled old woman ages ago. Instead, she has worked with her body, starting as soon as she was physically able—about six months after her sur-

Because of the fusion of the vertebrae in her neck, Margaret cannot do the regular stomach exercises. I have taught her to protect her neck, so that now she is so attuned to her body, she is able to do far more than one might expect and occasionally she will do one of the regular stomach exercises.

As soon as she feels pressure on her neck, she adjusts her position or stops. Sixty or so years ago, IdaMay, seen here with Scarlet, was an Earl Carroll's Vanities *showgirl. Still fit and in her mid-eighties, she works at her own pace and completes the class with everyone else.* ▲

gery—doing only what she could. Little by little she restored her body to good health. If she had been stiff and creaky and totally out of condition, she might have been severely injured by this recent fall.

"These exercises are saving my life," she swears. "I am strong and I'm flexible. I see people my age, even younger, deteriorating before my eyes. They have stooped shoulders and stumble and shuffle about, taking hesitant steps. I'm terrified of becoming that way. If I don't keep exercising, I know I will hunch over like a little old lady."

There is medical data to substantiate her observation about her own body. Inactivity does indeed speed the aging process. Often the limited movements and halting, painful steps of old age result from abuse or disuse begun in youth.

A dowager's hump and feeble posture are *not* the inevitable badges assigned by fate to women as they pass through middle age and beyond. In many ways, old age really *is* a state of mind. If you eat correctly and live and think like a young person, it stands to reason that you will look and feel young. You will move and walk with youthful ease. Some people are old and crotchety in their twenties; others are *never* old, despite what the calendar says.

The truth is that we all begin to age the moment we are born. Consequently, our bodies are ever aging. By the time we reach our forties, we begin to detect some real differences, most noticeably in our hair and skin, which change in color and texture. As our body chemistries change, we may notice some alteration in muscle tone, stiffness in our joints, and aches and pains in places we have never felt them before.

There is no need for a long explanation about cholesterol, triglycerides, and low-density/high-density lipoproteins, atherosclerotic plaques, arteriosclerosis, or even osteoporosis and calcium deficiencies, basal metabolism and cardiovascular fitness. You can keep abreast of the latest in medical data through current women's magazines and newspapers and, most important, by asking your doctor specific, candid questions about your feelings and about your body's changes.

Don't settle for a pat on the head and a "that's-a-good-girl" attitude from your family physician. Despite the natural changes our bodies experience—including the cessation of the menses and subsequent loss of estrogen in a woman's body—it is *not* normal or natural to creak through life after middle age.

The bottom line is this: The stooped, aching, feeble movements associated with the elderly can be avoided in most cases if we take care of our bodies while we are young. I am still paying the price for carrying around a heavy rucksack on my back for so long. If I don't exercise, I am in trouble.

There are some changes we must be aware of. Our eyesight often loses acuity. Bones often become brittle, making it all the more important that we keep our muscles in shape. Who wants to take a spill and break a hipbone? That can happen if one is out of shape and does not know *how* to fall.

Regular exercise is essential to maintaining minimim fitness, even more in the elderly than in the young. It is not enough to walk to the car or do your housework or gardening or play a round of golf or even tennis once a week. Make exercise a habit to forestall problems. As you exercise, you increase your energy level and, naturally, your body's potential. My older students can do as many as the younger students. I believe the older you get the more exercise your body needs.

The exercises Margaret does come from the same basic program I give to my younger students. As with anyone I teach, movements are adapted to what she can do. Sometimes she is able to do more, sometimes less. Because of her neck and back, I do not allow her to do the basic stomach exercises. Instead, she has devised her own version, using a pillow to raise her head and shoulders. Because of this, I refer you to the exercises for people with bad backs for your stomach exercises (see Chapter 17). As a rule, I do not give these to my older students until after their third class. If you have a pacemaker, they may be too strenuous for you.

For the sake of pictures, I had to insist that Margaret not show off. She does the exercises in the One-Hour Program usually better than women half her age. She can raise her leg to the *barre,* but since most people her age won't be able to do this, she is photographed using a lower ladder. I did not want her to intimidate someone less fit than she! I asked her to demonstrate this chapter because at her age and with her medical problems, she is more than aware of how gentle one must be with the body. This is the way she did the program before she built up her strength.

"I feel terrible if I don't exercise," she says. "The important thing is to stay active. Don't let yourself get past the point of no return, where your body can no longer move. So many people over fifty need a stick of dynamite to get them moving."

When someone seventy or so arrives in my class, the red carpet is laid out. Usually, they are mothers of my younger students. Most of them come to me demanding, very shyly, the same results as their children. I require that they tell me everything they are feeling, with every little movement. They are adorable! A sparkle comes to their eyes, especially after about the third hour, when they are beginning to keep up with the rest of the class and starting to see their skin becoming tight.

The stiffer a student is when I start working with her, the more I enjoy my work. Her body becomes very straight in an amazingly short amount of time. Eventually she walks very erect, and puts some teenagers to shame!

Older people are fun. They laugh a lot, and they are so gracious. It is very inspiring for everyone around them to see them work at their own pace, take a breather, and then keep on going. It doesn't bother me to see someone staring at herself in the mirror for five or ten minutes before getting back into the routine, because I know that it is just a matter of time before she will be able to keep up with the class and complete the entire hour's program without interruption.

The exercises photographed for this section are modifications of the One-Hour Program that everyone does. I see no reason to separate the age groups any more than the sexes! Study these pictures and read through the One-Hour Program, as well as the exercises for people with bad backs.

Work at your own pace, doing *what* you can, *when* you can, for as long as you can, until you are able to complete a program. Trust your body. It will let you know what you can and cannot do. When you feel you are ready, go to the One-Hour Program if you wish.

Note: *No jerking, no forcing. Every movement should be done in triple slow motion. Key word: gentleness.*
This is preparation for the warm-ups—stretching the spine. Sitting in a chair, you should lean your torso forward and stretch your arms out in front of you. Relax your body. ▶

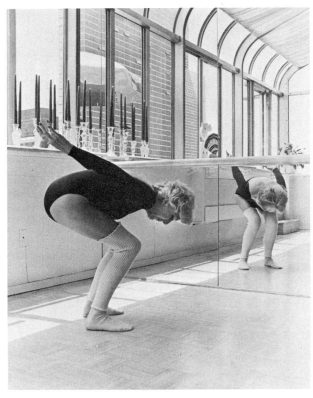

This basic warm-up is taken from the One-Hour Program. Stretch your arms up to the ceiling. Make your body feel 2 inches taller. Gently *bend your knees.* Keep your feet about a foot apart. Lower your arms, moving them high behind you. Return them to the side of your body and reach to the ceiling. Do 5. ▲

To stretch the waist, stand erect with your legs a foot to a foot-and-a-half apart. Put your left hand on your left hip, elbow bent. Tighten your behind and tip your pelvis upward as you reach your right arm high over your head. Gently *bend your torso to the left* with your right arm straight. Keep your behind tight and your pelvis upward. Keep your feet and hips even. Only bend over as far as you can to maintain proper balance. Gently move your torso back and forth a quarter of an inch. Start with 30 and build up to 50 on each side. ▼

Be very conscious of your body while doing this stretch for the spine and backs of the legs. With your feet a foot and a half apart, bend your body over toward the floor. Keep knees bent and put your hands above your knees for support. This way, your weight rests on your hands and thighs. Hold this position for a count of 20. Then move back up a quarter of an inch and down a quarter of an inch. Do 15 movements up and down. Never jerk or bounce. Do not move your torso more than a quarter of an inch. Without standing up, grab your inner knees with your hands. Gently move your body as if you are trying to push your head between your knees. Move a quarter of an inch at a time. Relax your legs and keep your knees flexed. Do 15 quarter-inch movements. ▼

Again, without straightening torso, gently *take both hands to outside of the right knee.* Make quarter-inch movements down with your head, shoulders, and upper body as though trying to put your head between your arms and your knee. Keep your legs relaxed and knees bent. Do 10 movements to the right, stretch torso out to the front, and then over to the left to do 10 on the left side. Then stand by rolling your spine upward until you are erect, using triple slow motion. ▲

If you do not have a barre, use the back of a sofa or sturdy chair, or even the kitchen counter. Use your imagination. The height of the barre is not important. Stand facing your barre, holding it with your hands at shoulder width. Stand on the balls of your feet with your heels together. Slightly bend your knees out to each side. Lower your body 1 or 2 inches and then return to the original position. Do not go lower. Do 10. Margaret is so fit that I had to hold her back for these pictures. Most older people have not worked their knees for quite a while, so special attention must be paid not to damage them. If you go lower than 2 inches, you will be putting too much pressure on the knee-joint complex at first. Hold on to the barre as much as you wish. Do 10. This works on your thighs, calves, ankles, and feet, building flexibility and strength. ▲

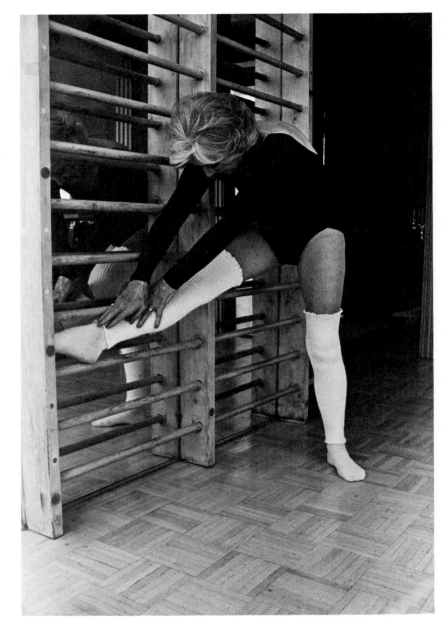

For this hamstring stretch, put your heel on a low table or chair, padding the table surface to protect your heel if necessary. Gently position your hands on any part of the leg except the knees. Move your torso a quarter inch toward your foot. Do not force. The body and legs should be relaxed, especially through the knees. Move torso in triple slow motion up and down a quarter of an inch, if you can. Do 20. Switch legs and repeat. With this, or any of the exercises you see in this chapter, if movement is difficult, don't move at all. Simply hold the position. ▲

Older people can adapt the exercises for the behind and hips that I teach in the One-Hour Program. Sit on the floor on your left cheek (far over on your left hip). Bend your left leg in front of your body and position your right leg on your right side, even with your right hip with the knee bent. Put both hands on the floor to the left of

your left knee for balance. Relax your torso. Gently *lift your right knee and foot off the floor* and with half-inch movements, push the right knee to the back and then return to the original position. Keep hips even. Do 15 to 20 on each side if possible the first time. As you feel stronger, increase to 30, and then to 50. ◄

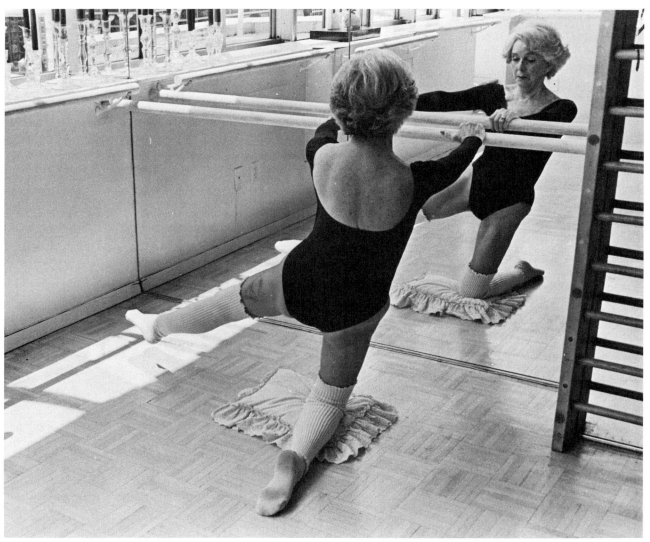

Kneel on a cushion in front of whatever you are using or barre, *arms extended outward.* Grasp barre at shoulder width and lean back so that your elbows are straight. Keeping your hips even, extend your left leg out to the side. Tighten your behind muscles and tip your pelvis up. Relax and round your shoulders. Gently *lift your left leg up and down, moving only 2 inches off the floor.* Even if you can't lift your foot, keep trying. Talk to your leg. You'll be able to do it sooner or later. Do 10 on each side. If you have knee problems, ask your doctor if you should do this. You may also try doing it while standing, as long as you bend a little the knee of the leg you are standing on, following same directions. ▲

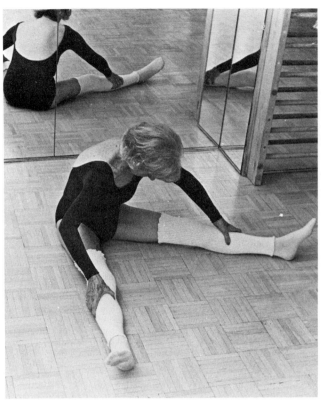

To stretch the inner thigh, sit on the floor and spread your legs as far as you can without forcing or losing balance. Relax your body and legs. Bend your torso forward and place your hands on your legs as close to your feet as is comfortable. Bend your elbows and hold this position for a count of 30. Then move gently up and down a quarter of an inch. Do 30. If your legs don't straighten, bend your knees. ▲

Give your spine and hamstrings a thorough stretch. Lie on your back, resting your head on a small pillow to support your neck. Margaret must use a pillow to protect her neck because of her fusion. Bend your legs at the knee and bring up to your chest. Clasp your hands in back of your knees, calves, or ankles—whichever is more comfortable, and ease your knees toward your chest. This should not be a pulling or jerking motion. Either hold or gently move toward your chest a quarter of an inch and then go back to your original position. Do 20. Gently bend your knees and return your legs to the floor. Take a breather before continuing with the next exercise. ▼

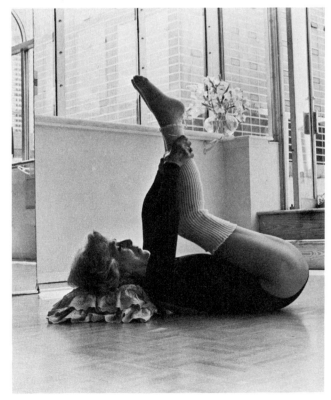

To further stretch the spine, as well as the thighs and stomach muscles, lie on your back with your hands at your sides. Rest your head on a pillow to protect your head and neck. Tighten your behind and push your pelvis off the floor. Gently push the pelvis up a quarter of an inch higher, then lower. Do 20. Keep your arms, neck, and feet relaxed. ▶

All I ask of my students is that they do as much as they can when exercising. Unlike programs where you are expected to keep up or drop out, I encourage students to rest when they feel tired, then continue when they are rested.

Until your body is ready, you may look a little awkward doing some of the exercises. That doesn't bother me a bit, as I would rather look a little awkward now and have a fabulous figure later on. ▲

CHAPTER TWENTY

Overcoming Problems

An Arabian proverb says:

He who has health has hope;
and he who has hope has everything.

While health can be a relative matter, I certainly agree that hope is the fuel that keeps us going. Hope is the heart of survival.

My personal hope kept me alive throughout my travels. It propelled me as I learned to exercise through pain to strengthen my own body.

One beautiful young woman who had polio as a child proved to me again that even someone with apparent physical disabilities can exercise and become fit. A bride of only a few months, she came to my studio with her handsome husband. As is typical of people who are confined to wheelchairs or who must walk with crutches, her upper body was muscular, though lean. Her lower limbs and buttocks shook as she dragged her feet and legs along the floor, moving across the room on aluminum crutches.

I had told them when they contacted me about classes that I had no previous experience with the physically disabled. My technique comes strictly from common sense and practical personal experience. Knowing this, they still came in for private lessons. As the husband told me, they wanted the lower part of her body to become strong and firm. They heard of my program from students and had seen the incredibly fast results.

I must admit that I was nervous. I honestly did not know the extent of her paralysis or what, if anything, I would be able to do for her. And I didn't know what they expected of me. Surely this woman had been given physical therapy through the years. I had to hold back tears when her husband took her crutches and she sank to the floor, gripping the *barre* with both hands.

I positioned her body for the behind exercises—the same as in the One-Hour Program. Then I showed her how to do them.

I don't know how, but she struggled until she was able to move just a little. When she protested, she looked to her husband for support.

Imagine my shock when he told her to quit being a crybaby and to get on with the exercises! "I love you too much to let you be a complete cripple," he said. She continued. Slowly. Deliberately. She did only what she could.

I was a wreck!

This gorgeous creature took two private lessons with me before she and her husband moved out West. They taped a class so that she would be able to continue working with her body. Even after these two sessions, I learned later, she began to experience muscle tone she never thought possible.

A few months after they left New York, the husband called me to say that she was *still* exercising and that she looked and felt magnificent! He also told me that she did not drag her feet as much as before. Of course, she will always need crutches to get about, but he told me her behind was already getting very tight.

To this day, I cannot understand how she did the exercises. I don't know where this daring couple is today, but I thank them for reminding me in two short hours what determination and willpower can accomplish.

Scoliosis and lupus have limited Tara's flexibility, but have not stifled her determination. She cannot raise her arms in back to do this warming-up stretch for the underarms and pectoral areas, but she does them as well as she can. Her thumbs are pointed upward and her arms rolled over for maximum stretch. As with all of my exercises, each movement is slow and gentle. Notice how one leg is shorter than the other—the result of her back condition. ▲

Another student who is an inspiration to me and to my other students is Tara. Her physical problems are mammoth, but her attitude and emotional strength are empowering to all of us.

In her mid-thirties, Tara has scoliosis so severely that one leg is noticeably shorter than the other. She has a congenital calcium deficiency and milk allergy, which, as a child, affected bone development.

For twelve years, Tara has been treated with cortisone for systemic lupus erythematosus (lupus), a chronic inflammatory and connective tissue disease that involves the vital organs and autoimmune system. It is manifest by extremely swollen joints that become red, hot, and stiff during periods of inflammation.

Despite medical conditions that most of us would consider to be debilitating, Tara has incredible spunk. She has found that if she does not exercise, she loses mobility. Consequently, she makes a concerted effort to improve her body potential. For a while she worked with a chiropractor who helped her to see the wisdom in giving up high heels.

"I was in more pain because I insisted on being in style," Tara laughs. "He helped me see how silly that was and made me stop wearing heels altogether."

Initially, Tara came to me because she had heard that this program was good for people with weak or damaged knees. She *labored* with the exercises, doing the most her body would allow. For her first six classes she could not raise her legs off the floor to do the Open & Close. In very little time she found benefits she never expected from this, or any program. Her lower back is stronger; she has improved flexibility, and now has physical strength that far surpasses the norm for people with her problems.

All this because she does what she can—her best.

Tara does this advanced exercise for her hips and behind because she can't kneel. I don't teach this to most students because it takes so much control. Tara is very conscious of what her body can and cannot do. It may seem that she is doing this and other exercises incorrectly. Not true. She is doing what is correct for her. She wears specially-fitted running shoes even while exercising for balance. ▲

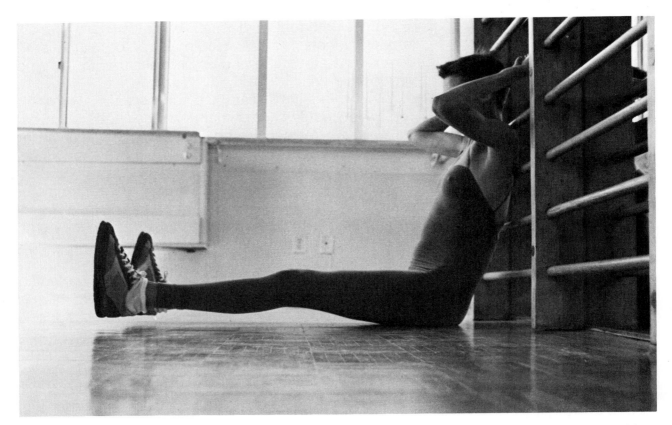

This is possibly the most difficult exercise I teach, yet, because she has such strength in her abdominal muscles, Tara is able to do it with relative ease. She sits with her behind 5 inches from the wall and rests her upper back and shoulders against it. Tara's lack of mobility limits her reach, so she works against the ladder, clasping the rung just above her head with both hands. Because she cannot bend her knees from the starting position to achieve a higher leg lift, Tara merely raises both legs off the floor as high as she can and opens and closes them about an inch off the floor. She can do as many as my advanced students without problems. ▲

—— CHAPTER TWENTY-ONE ——

The Advanced Program

Most of my students are not even aware that I have introduced them to a program of advanced exercises until they are well into it. When I see that someone has acquired enough strength and stamina—which is usually after the fourth or fifth class—I give her some new movements to integrate into her program. It may be a new way to tip the pelvis or turn the leg, something subtle that transforms the basic exercises into more powerful, advanced exercises.

The progression from the One-Hour Program to the Advanced Program is a gradual, very individual move. Unless a student demonstrates the physical ability to do more, I keep her at the basic level. I do not compare one student with another, nor do I have a timetable that says that by the fifth class everyone should be doing the advanced behind exercises, or that by the seventh everyone *must* do the advanced stretches. I do not permit my students to begin an exercise unless I have evidence that their bodies are prepared for it.

Do not start these exercises until you have completely mastered the One-Hour Program. You are looking at some very potent movements and your body *must* be ready for them. One advanced stomach or behind movement, for example, is equivalent to twenty of the comparable beginners' movement. These exercises may *look* the same as those in the One-Hour Program. Don't be fooled: They are the same, but with some very precise, subtle changes. If you follow the directions correctly, you will immediately feel the differences.

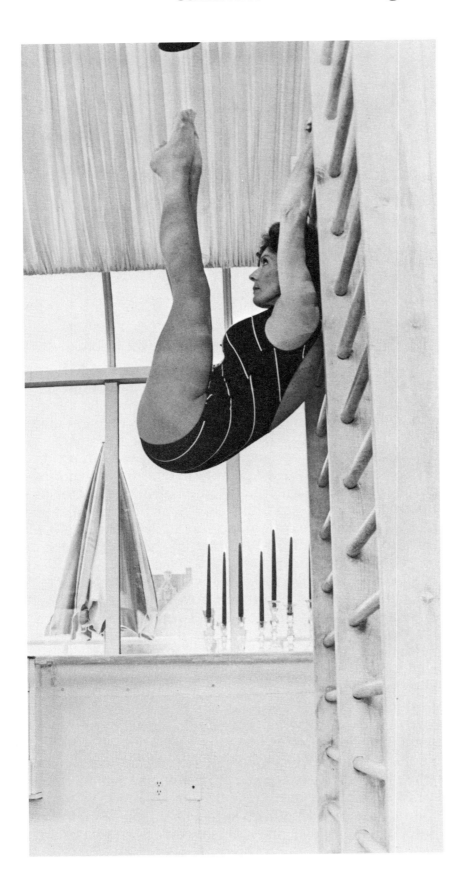

This hanging leg lift is a test in body strength. Do not attempt this unless you have access to a studio ladder, such as I have, a chinning bar, or a gymnasium with proper equipment that can support your weight. You also must have tremendous strength in your wrists, shoulders, and arms to do it safely. It takes incredible abdominal strength and, once mastered, this exercise can be expanded to include opening and closing your legs as you hang. Even now I can only do 20 sequences at this height. ◄

All of the students you saw in the One-Hour Program are beginners, with fewer than three classes at the time their pictures were taken. They demonstrate how to do the exercises quite properly, but they are not ready to go to the maximum level with them. By the time they have mastered the One-Hour Program, they will have the strength and flexibility to execute every exercise I do in this Advanced Program.

The challenge of this upper level plan is another reason to move on. It is a magnificent feeling to master one set of body moves and then reach out even further toward the mastery of even more difficult movements. Ultimately, you will have integrated the two levels of challenge into one totally personal program that takes the same amount of time.

Yet another obvious reason to advance to a more difficult program is boredom. Exercise, I am the first to admit, can be monotonous and boring. If you can introduce some variety into your body work, you will find the time passing like a breeze.

Because of the high level of control needed to do these advanced movements, you will feel and see results every time you do them. I show you how to alter the basic program into advanced movements, explaining in detail how to do the new, more difficult, advanced level. When you are certain you are ready for them, move ahead.

WARMING UP *Stand erect with your feet 12 to 15 inches apart and stretch arms and body upward. Tip your pelvis up, tightening your behind. Bend your upper body forward, arms out in front of you, as though reaching for something just out of reach in front of you. Knees are bent. Continue bending the knees and leaning forward; bring arms up behind you. Return to starting position. Repeat 15 times, keeping your knees relaxed.* ▶

FOR TIGHT UNDERARMS
Again, drawing from the One-Hour Program, the underarm tightener begins by standing erect, feet slightly apart, pelvis tipped forward. Stretch your arms out to the sides at shoulder level. Roll arms over and, keeping your arms straight and high, reach behind you as if you were trying to make your hands and shoulder blades meet. Hold head and shoulders up and back. Move arms only a half inch at a time, back and forth behind you. Keep arms as high as you can. Do 100. To learn better balance, do it while standing on one foot. When you reach 50, change feet. ▼

WAIST STRETCH   *Reach one arm up and over your head and stretch as far to the opposite side as you can. Rest the other hand on your thigh. Remember to keep this arm out and bent to support your lower back. Notice how straight and even my hips are and how I keep my pelvis tipped upward. Most of my students can stretch over much further than I can because of my back problems. Even so, I am 4 inches smaller in the waist than when I was a teenager. Keep raised elbows straight. Do 100 in each direction.* ▲

178

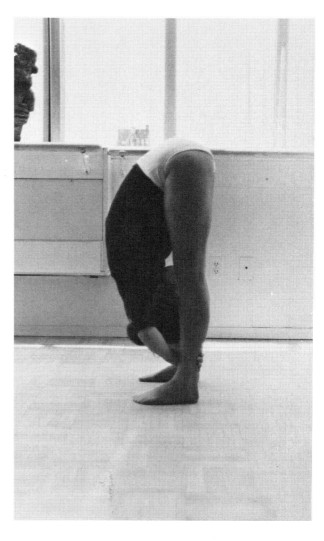

THE ADVANCED STRETCH
From that position, clasp hands, fingers straight, and bend straight over. Keep your arms behind your back. Do not tighten your knees. Slowly put your nose to your knees and move your arms as close to the floor as possible. Hold for a count of 20. This is to be done in triple *slow motion. Do not lock knees. Keep legs relaxed.* ▲

Without straightening up, move your arms down your leg and clasp your ankles from the inside. You probably will have to slip your feet apart a few inches to do this. If you are not ready to grasp your legs from the inside, hold on from the outside for a slow count of 20. ▲

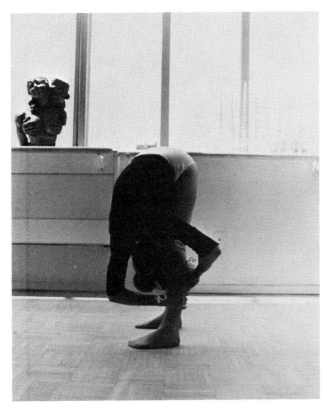

Turn torso to one side as low as you can. Grasp your leg from the outside, keeping your elbows bent out. You can do this with your feet together or apart. Try to move your head past your knee, between it and your outside elbow. Keep both hips even. Do not lock your knees. Do 20. Do not straighten up. Instead, gently move to other side and repeat. ▲

From that position, still keeping legs relaxed, move your hands to the floor, fingers facing each other. Bend your elbows. Gently move your torso a half inch lower and move up and down 20 times from there. If you are unable to move, hold for a slow count of 20. Return to a standing position by curling your shoulders upward as you straighten your spine. This powerful combination stretches your hamstrings, calves, shoulder blades, and lower back. It works wonders on your balance. ▼

FOR THE STOMACH #1
Begin as you would to do the first stomach exercise in the One-Hour Program. Pull your upper torso upward, keeping your shoulders rounded and your elbows bent outward. Your body and legs should be relaxed. Let go of your legs and gently move up and down from that point. Notice how high my shoulders are. An inch higher and I would be using my back muscles. The object is to work on the stomach and abdominal muscles. Do 100. ▲

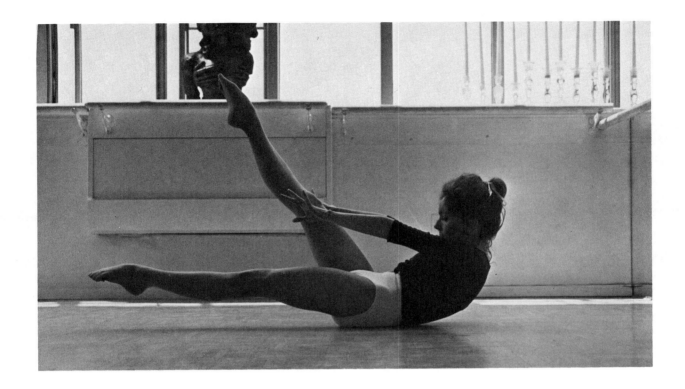

FOR THE STOMACH #2 *Lie flat on the floor. Lift your left leg 6 inches off the floor and raise your right leg perpendicular to your body. Clasp your hands behind your raised knee. Pull your upper torso off the floor, rounding your shoulders and keeping your head pushed forward. Let go of your knee and, without letting your shoulders fall back, move up and down a half inch in both directions. Do 100 with each leg.* ▲

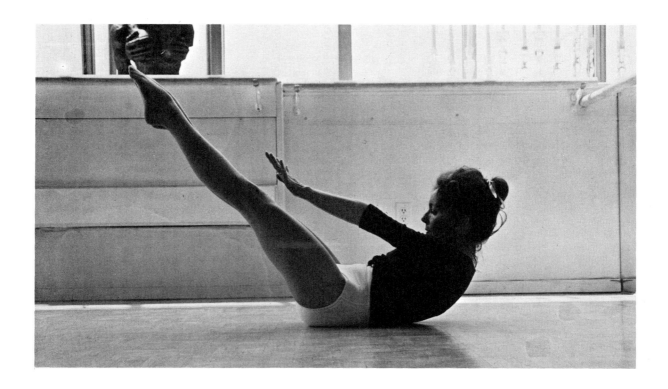

FOR THE STOMACH #3
Rounding out the stomach series is this precise move, done with both legs up. You can move legs lower than this, but be sure that you do not let the small of your back come off the floor. The lower the legs, the more the back will try to take over for your stomach muscles. Be sure your stomach muscles are strong enough to hold this lower position of your legs. As explained in the One-Hour Program, grab your outer thighs to pull your upper body off the floor. Push the small of your back into the floor. Let go of your legs and extend arms out straight. Start to lower your legs without letting your back muscles take over. If you feel pressure, that is your signal that your stomach muscles are not strong enough to lower your legs further. You must raise them to a position comfortable for your back. Do 100. ▲

THE ADVANCED STOMACH EXERCISE #1 *Sit up with both knees bent, feet flat on the floor, head and shoulders rounded forward, and pelvis tipped upward. Scoot forward with your bottom so that you are not sitting on your tailbone. Your palms will be on your knees and your elbows out as far as possible. Tuck your head between your arms, resting your forehead on your knees.* ◄

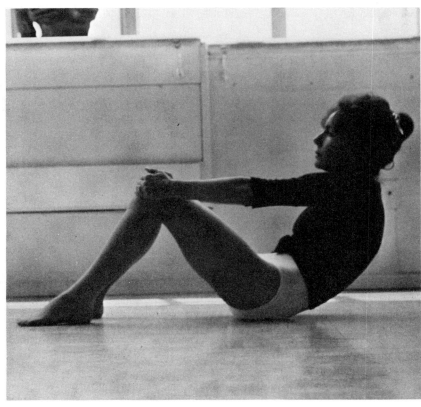

Tighten your behind and, without straightening your back, continue to tip your pelvis upward like a scoop. Your back will automatically stay rounded as long as you just roll your pelvis toward your waist while holding your knees until your arms are straight. ◄

Let go of your knees. Do not let your torso move. Keep your pelvis curled up and your shoulders rounded. Gracefully raise your arms upward, even with your ears. If you feel your feet coming off the floor, straighten your legs a little in front of you. ▶

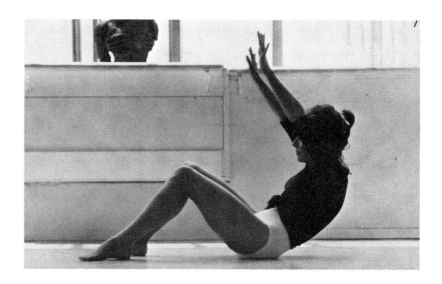

Hold that position without letting your upper body roll backward. Slowly lower your arms until your fingertips touch the floor. Gracefully raise and lower your arms 10 times without letting your body roll back. Breathe easily, normally. This is excellent for learning balance. ▶

Without moving your body, return your hands to your knees. Arms should be straight and back rounded. Your pelvis should be tipped upward. Without altering your position, take a breather. Curl pelvis up still more, lower your body a little further, and repeat, moving your arms up and down 10 times. To complete exercise, slowly lower your shoulders to the floor vertebra by vertebra. You will feel the strength and power of the abdominal muscles doing all the work. ▶

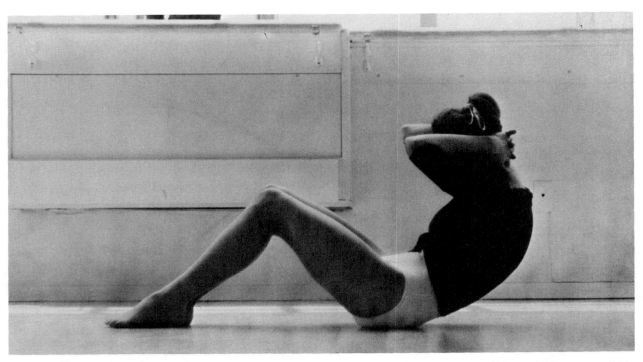

THE ADVANCED STOMACH EXERCISE #2 *From the same starting position as the previous exercise, clasp your hands behind your head and lean your head forward, your chin on your chest, and your forehead on* *your knees. Lower your body to the floor by curling your pelvis up even further, using your stomach muscles to ease yourself back, one vertebra at a time. The closer your feet are to your behind, the more your stomach will work and* *you will have to tip your pelvis higher to roll back. Do this extremely slowly with control. Once is enough, if you do this correctly.* ▲

FOR THE LEGS #1 *Face the barre and hold it with both hands. Keep shoulders straight. Go up on your toes (not the balls of your feet), heels together. Move your pelvis upward a half inch farther than you think you can and then back. Go down 2 inches lower. Repeat this process 3 times and then reverse directions until you are back at your starting position. Do not stick out behind.* ◄

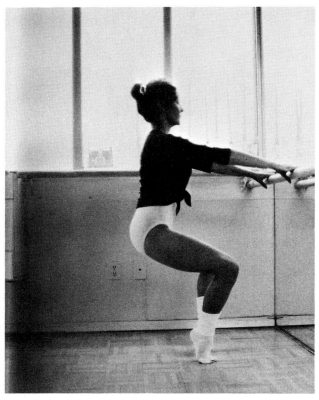

FOR THE LEGS #2 *The second exercise for the legs begins like the first: on your toes, heels together, holding the barre with both hands. Lower your body 10 to 12 inches, slowly and gently, then return to the top position. Repeat 20 times. Rest as needed.* ▲

FOR THE LEGS #3 *Start in the same position as in the One-Hour Program. Rest your right heel on the barre. Fold your hands across your ankle. Keep your hips even. Do not lock the knee of the leg you're standing on. Stretch your head and body forward. When you can't go any further, hold, letting your head go down further, either resting it on your foot or letting it go to the left. Stretch and relax. Count to 50.* ▼

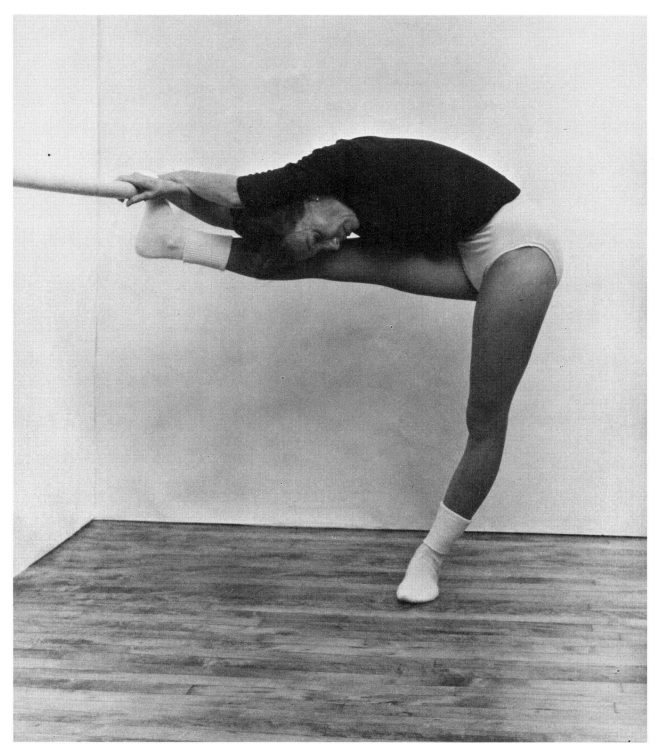

FOR THE LEGS #4 *Place the arch of your foot on the barre, holding your hands on each side of your foot. Gently scoot your standing foot toward the barre and cross your hands (as in the drawing) over your foot. Gently straighten the bent leg. Bend elbows and put your head between your leg and arm. Straighten your leg to increase the stretch. Gently move your body back and forth—very slowly, please—50 times.*
IMPORTANT: *If you have a tendency toward sciatica, do not do this exercise.* ▲

189

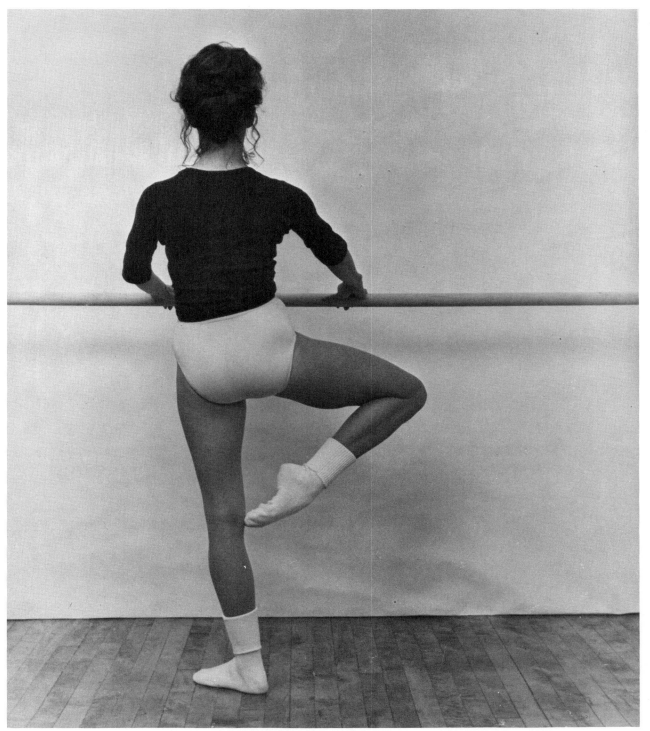

ADVANCED LEG EXERCISE
This graceful leg movement is fantastic for toning and shaping your legs while working on your balance. It is rooted in my ballet training, as you may have guessed. Face the barre, holding it gently with both hands. Bend your right leg up and out to one side, pointing your toe toward the knee of your upright leg. (Don't lock your knees.) ▲

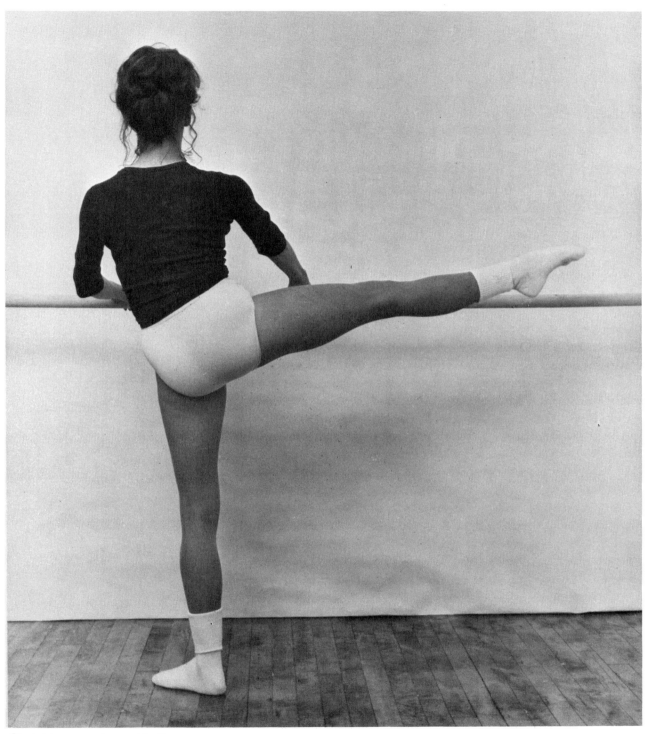

Straighten your leg out to the side without dropping it to the floor. Relax your shoulders. Keep your body erect, head up. ▲

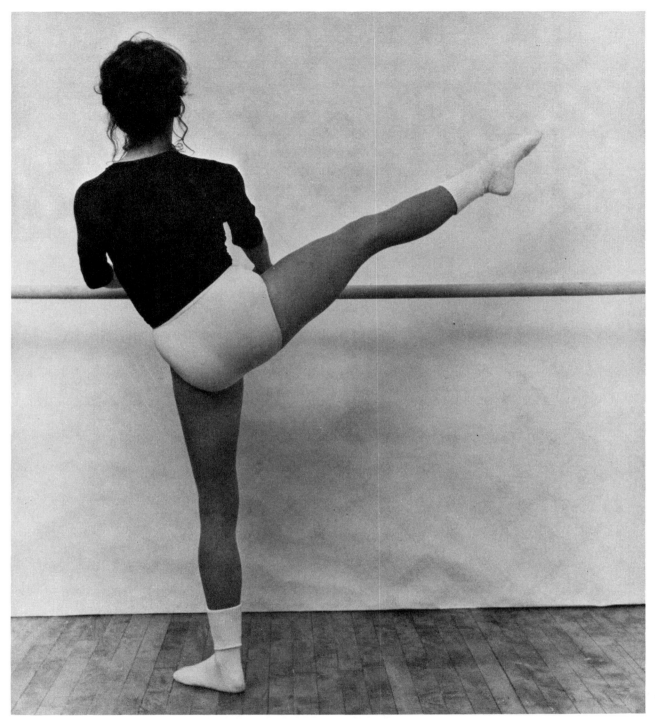

Bend your knee again and raise your leg at least 1 inch higher. Straighten your leg at the higher level. Bend and raise leg still higher, until you can reach this height. Then slowly lower leg to the floor. Do 10 times with each leg. ▲

FOR THE BEHIND AND HIPS
#1 *The first of the exercises for the behind and hips is straight from the One-Hour Program. Notice how the left hip is rolled as far forward as possible, much more than in the basic program, and is even with*

the right hip. You should be able to keep your back straight. Don't lean over. The left knee is even with the left hip, but about 4 inches from the floor. Knee and foot are level. Move knee ever so gently a half inch to an

inch back, then return to the side, even with the hip. Do 100 with each leg. Keep behind tight and pelvis tipped up. ▲

FOR THE BEHIND AND HIPS

#2 *This behind exercise starts in the same way as #1, but with the left leg straight out to the side. Roll the hip forward. Keep behind tight, pelvis tipped up, and foot turned into the floor.*

Try to get your leg as high off the floor as possible. Sit erect

with your hip rolled forward. If you are doing everything correctly, you won't be able to lift your extended leg more than 3 inches off the floor. Move leg up and down, a half inch in each direction, slowly and gently. Do 100 with each leg. ◀

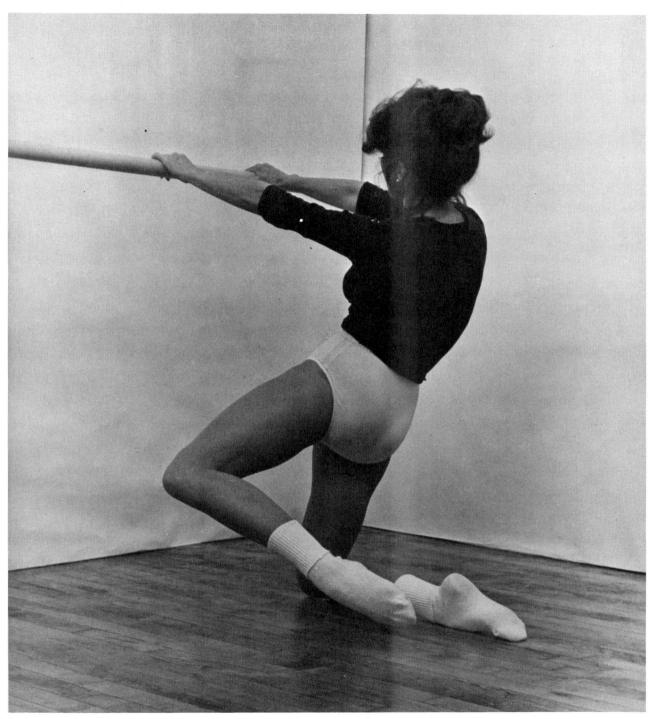

FOR THE BEHIND AND HIPS
#3 *If you do this kneeling exercise for the behind and hips correctly, this is as high as you will be able to lift your foot off the floor. Keeping both hips even, tightening your behind, and tipping the pelvis up, round* *your shoulders. Lean to the right to take weight off kneecaps. Raise your left knee out to the side, concentrating on keeping your hips even. Turn your knee to the ceiling. Notice how it is higher than my foot. Also notice how straight* *my lower back is and how rounded my shoulders. Move back and forth in tiny, precise movements, a half inch to an inch in each direction, but not in front of your hips. Only bring knee even with hip. Do 100 with each leg.* ▲

FOR THE BEHIND AND HIPS
#4 *Kneel facing the barre, holding it with hands at shoulder width. If possible, stretch right leg straight out to the right. Keep lower back straight and shoulders rounded, hips even. Lean your body to the left, pulling your leg to your body without bending knee. You can see how far by noting the tape mark on the floor. This takes your weight off your left kneecap. Keep foot turned to the floor. Tighten behind. Tip your pelvis up. Then lift your right leg off the floor 2 inches— or as high as you can—and move up and down. Do 100 with each leg. Keep your leg relaxed without locking your knee.* ◀

ADVANCED BEHIND AND HIP EXERCISE #1 *This advanced exercise is never taught until a student has had 4 or 5 hours in class and their bodies are strong enough to be in control. It only* looks *simple! Stand with your feet together, facing the* barre. *Raise your left knee to the side, turning it upward and pointing your foot behind you. Tighten your behind and curl your pelvis up. Lean your shoulders toward your raised leg. This keeps pressure off your back and helps you to keep your pelvis up. Keep hips even. Move your leg to the back in tiny, precise movements, keeping your knees up. Do 100 on each side. Do not lock right knee. This and #2 are substitutes for the kneeling exercises in the One-Hour Program if you have bad knees or bruise easily.* ▶

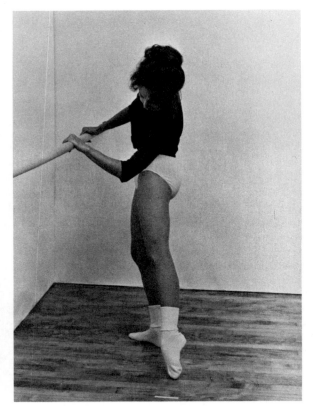

ADVANCED BEHIND AND HIP EXERCISE #2 *As you stand facing the* barre, *keep your hips even and your right knee bent just a little. Take your left leg straight out to the left side, still keeping your hips even and your back straight. Head is up, shoulders relaxed.* ▲

Bring your left leg toward your right foot. Lean your body to the right, keeping your behind tight and your pelvis tipped upward. Notice how far I have brought my leg from the marker. Lean your shoulders over to the left, relax.

Then lift your leg up and down. If you are standing properly, you won't be able to get your foot more than 5 inches off the floor. This is especially true if your hips are even and pelvis is curled up. Do 100 on each side. ▲

OPEN & CLOSE *Sit against the wall with your behind 3 to 6 inches from the baseboard and your shoulders against the wall. Grasp the* barre—*or whatever you are using—with both hands. If you feel you want to stretch your spine further, lean your chin forward. With your legs together, bend your knees and raise your legs up in a jackknife in front of your body. Straighten your legs, keeping them high, and slowly open and close. Do not lock knees. The higher you raise them and the wider you open them, the more your thigh muscles will tighten. Do 100—4 sets of 25, if necessary.* ▶

STRETCH #1 *Spread your legs as far as you can. Point your toes but keep them relaxed. Stretch your arms forward and lean your upper body forward as far as you can.*

Move forward from there gently until your chest is on the floor. Then stretch to each side, resting head and arms on leg. Do 50 in each direction. ▲

STRETCH #2 *With legs together sit erect. Reach your arms out behind you, palms together. Lean forward, feet flexed, stretching over to rest your head on your knees with your arms up in back. Hold for a count of 25. Do not force.* ▲

STRETCH #3 *This is a beautiful hamstring stretch. Lie flat on the floor, back and shoulders relaxed. Bend your right knee to your chest then straighten leg upward. Clasp your right leg gently with both hands at the ankle and ease it softly toward your chest. Keep your arms relaxed, elbows bent outward. Gently bring leg toward chest. Relax. Do 50 times with each leg. ▲*

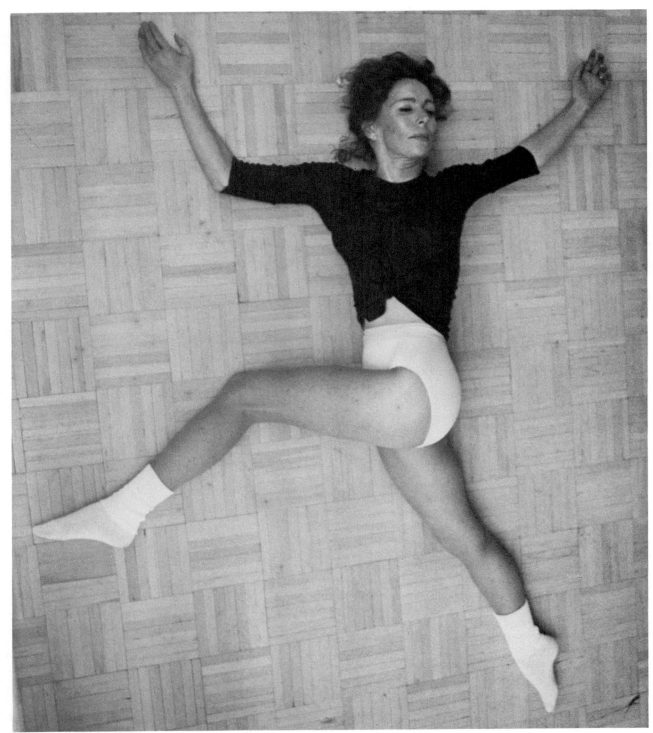

STRETCH #4 *For someone with the least hint of back pain, this could be called the best stretch. Lie flat on the floor, arms bent at shoulder level. Keep elbows on the floor. Raise your left leg up and cross over* *to the right side, as though you are trying to touch your right elbow with your left knee. Keep your right leg on the floor. The higher you can take your knee to your arms and the straighter you can keep your right leg, the* *more stretch you will feel through your pectorals, your spine, between your shoulder blades, even your sacrum, hamstrings, and thighs. Hold for a count of 40 on each side.* ▲

STRETCH #5 *This is a grown-up version of the split everybody learned in phys. ed. or dancing school. I give it to some of my advanced students and do it myself for flexibility, letting hand rest on leg for balance. My students like to do it because they feel like gymnasts! It's a superb stretch for your thighs. Do not force. Hold for a count of 30.* ▲

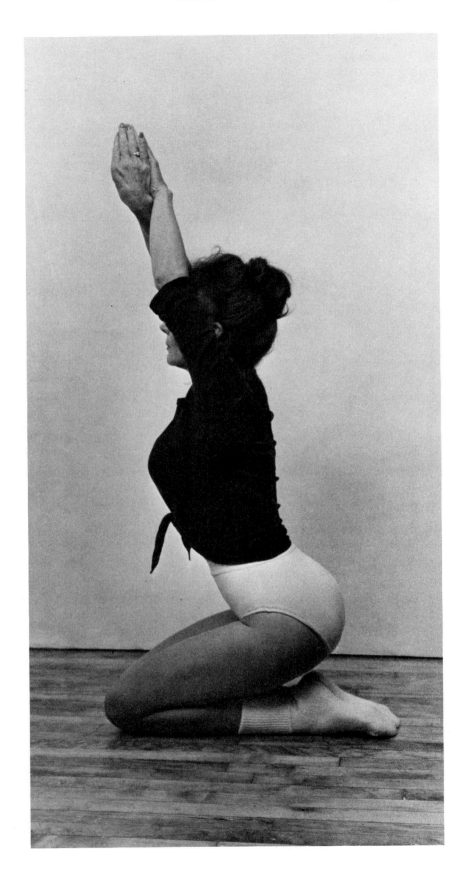

PELVIC ROTATIONS *As with the Scoop, Pelvic Rotations are wonderful for the pelvis and lower back and they give your thighs a wonderful stretch. Sit on your heels, hands clasped and arms stretched high over your head. Raise your body 3 inches from your heels and move your hip to the right. Now curl pelvis up in front, then over to the left, and finally back to complete the circle. Move only your pelvis (like a belly dancer) without dropping your behind to your heels. Make large, smooth circles. Do 20 clockwise and 20 counterclockwise. For variety, you can move your hips and pelvis in a Figure 8.* ◄

THE PELVIC SCOOP *The Pelvic Scoop increases flexibility in the pelvic area and tightens the inner thighs and the abdominal muscles. Kneel with your arms over your head. Stretch your body and arms high. Then aim your behind down to your heels. Curl your pelvis upward like a scoop and tighten your behind muscles. Keep your knees together. Continue tipping your pelvis upward, lifting your body up to the starting position. Do 20.* ▶

THE THIGH STRETCH *This powerful stretch gently stretches your pectorals, thighs, neck, stomach muscles, as well as your spine. Kneel, sitting on your heels. Put your hands behind you on the floor behind your feet. Relax your neck and let your head fall back toward the floor. Tighten your behind and curl your pelvis upward, raising your behind off your heels. Push pelvis up as high as you think you can and then push up even higher. Relax. Do 20 times.* ▲

THE INNER THIGH SQUEEZE *Do the Inner Thigh Squeeze, as taught in the One-Hour Program, as you have already learned. Hold for a count of 300. See the photos in the One-Hour Program to refresh your memory on how to do this.*

MY DEEPEST APPRECIATION
TO MY STUDENTS WHO ARE
PICTURED ON THESE PAGES

Faye Beckerman
Shira Boardman
Ellen M. Godowitz
Audrey Hagemailer
Tobi Himmel
Susan Kent
Kelle Kerr
Harvey Koeppel
Lisa McElroy
Lynne Meena
Jane Pinckney Middleton
Lane Middleton
Page Middleton
Janet Milazzo
IdaMay Otto
Hernando Perez
Margaret Pfeiffer Pinckney
Karl S. Sabo
Melanie Schor
Ellen Sthika
Harry Sloofman
Carolyn Smith
Katie Studley
Tara Terrell
Neal Thompson
Anna Tipton
Mary Tipton
Janet Valente Ben-Ami
Susan Wallace

QUESTIONS AND ANSWERS ABOUT

Callanetics

What makes this exercise program more effective than others?
The answer is Callanetics.

What is Callanetics?
It is exercises that activate the body's deepest, largest muscles.

What does Callanetics do for you?
If properly applied, these exercises can make an appreciable difference in your figure in 2 hours, a substantial difference in 4 hours, a dramatic difference in 5 to 7 hours, and a spectacular difference in 8 to 10 hours.

Where is the proof of this claim?
The proof is in the unretouched photos of this book. The remaining proof comes from doing it yourself and seeing the changes in your own body.

Can Callanetics cure any figure problem?
Callanetics will melt fat off buttocks and hips, flatten the tummy, stretch the neck, firm the chin, lift and tighten the rear and bust, slim inner thighs and legs, firm the underarms, and give you the perfect figure nature intended you to have.

Is Callanetics safe?
Callanetics is so safe that even eighty-year-olds can do these exercises.

Why is this so?
The deep muscles are activated by small and delicate movements consistently applied. There is no sudden jerking, no hard impact which can cause harm to the body, as sometimes happens in other forms of exercise.

What are these deep muscles and why are they so important?
The large underlying muscles are the ones that support the other, outlying muscles. By activating these major muscles you go directly to the source of a good figure.

Do you have to diet as well as exercise?
No. A person who is 10 to 15 pounds overweight can pull in so that his or her clothing is *two* sizes smaller without shedding a pound. If you do lose 10 pounds it will look like 20.